D0462206

DIAGNOSIS: SCHIZOPHRENIA

DIAGNOSIS:

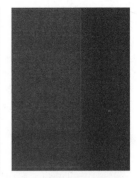

SCHIZOPHRENIA

Columbia University Press
New York

A COMPREHENSIVE
RESOURCE FOR
CONSUMERS, FAMILIES,
AND HELPING
PROFESSIONALS

RACHEL MILLER and SUSAN E. MASON

SECOND EDITION

Columbia University Press

Publishers Since 1893

New York   Chichester, West Sussex

Copyright © 2011 Columbia University Press

All rights reserved

Library of Congress Cataloging-in-Publication Data

Diagnosis: schizophrenia : a comprehensive resource for consumers, families, and helping professionals / [edited by] Rachel Miller and Susan E. Mason. — 2nd ed.

p.   cm.

Includes index.

ISBN 978-0-231-15040-8 (cloth : alk. paper) — ISBN 978-0-231-15041-5 (pbk.) — ISBN 978-0-231-52102-4 (electronic)

1. Schizophrenia—Case studies. I. Miller, Rachel, M.S.W. II. Mason, Susan Elizabeth. III. Title.

RC514.D44   2011

616.89'8—dc22   2010005500

References to Internet Web sites (URLs) were accurate at the time of writing. Neither the author nor Columbia University Press is responsible for URLs that may have expired or changed since the manuscript was prepared.

CONTENTS

Foreword to the Second Edition

When Rachel Miller and Susan Mason asked me to update the foreword for the second edition of *Diagnosis: Schizophrenia*, my first reaction was to ask, "Can you just use what I wrote in 1999?" They graciously said yes, and we agreed that the foreword to the first edition should be included in the present volume. But the ten years since I wrote those words have seen important advances in our understanding of schizophrenia and specific therapeutics available for people early in the course of their illness, as well as in our views of how and when to engage patients and their families.

The second edition therefore includes new information about the brain and schizophrenia, genetics, and childhood-onset schizophrenia. In addition, new medications are available, and these and their side effects are considered. Perhaps the most important changes are in sections that deal with coping with side effects of medication like weight gain, help with substance abuse and smoking, understanding delusions, dealing with violent thoughts and feelings, and negotiating the system of benefits for medication and Medicaid.

In addition to the advances in understanding schizophrenia and the guidance that has developed over that past decade, publication of the second edition of *Diagnosis: Schizophrenia* comes at a time when the National Institute of Mental Health (NIMH) has initiated a major research effort designed to change both perceptions and outcomes of schizophrenia. RAISE—Recovery After an Initial Schizophrenia Episode—is a large-scale research project initiated by the NIMH in the summer of 2009. It will develop and test innovative and coordinated intervention approaches in the early stages of the illness, when individuals may be most responsive to treatment. For more information and updates on this initiative, you can go to the NIMH RAISE Project Page on the NIMH Web site: www. nimh.nih.gov/health/topics/schizophrenia/raise/index.shtml.

The first edition has been successful beyond our hopes for a volume that built on the experiences of patients at a single clinic; over 20,000 copies have been sold—reaching patients and families at treatment settings and in communities throughout the United States and beyond. In addition to the audience for which it was designed, psychiatry residents and other clinicians new to schizophrenia treatment have found that it is a valuable tool. I have bought a number of copies myself to distribute. Understanding the perspective of patients and their families as they first encounter the health system and trying to see both the experience of the illness and the clinical world through their eyes can be invaluable.

So, the recommendation for *Diagnosis: Schizophrenia*, second edition is much the same as for the first edition. Read it cover to cover or check the table of contents or index if you need some specific information, and remember that just as individuals change over time, so will our understanding of schizophrenia and of the ways to help individuals and their families cope and grow.

Nina Schooler, Ph.D.

Professor of Psychiatry and Behavioral Sciences

SUNY Downstate Medical Center

Brooklyn, New York

Foreword

In 1966, when I was a student, I attended my first case conference in a psychiatric hospital. Sitting around the table were the psychiatrist who was the director of a 150-bed division in this large urban hospital, the patient's treating psychiatrist, and other members of the treatment team: a social worker, a clinical psychologist, a clinical psychology intern, and other students. The patient we were discussing was a young man who was experiencing his first hospitalization, and everyone seemed to agree that the evidence pointed to a diagnosis of schizophrenia. When the discussion was over, all eyes turned to the director. He nodded sagely and said something like: "This is a very nice young man. We should not give him such a terrible diagnosis at this time. When he comes back the next time . . . that will be time enough. Now, let us find another diagnosis." There was a universal nod of agreement, and then the group found another diagnosis.

In 1999 I attended another case conference, this time for a young woman who was experiencing her first hospitalization. The patient was interviewed by the head of the psychiatry department, with staff and trainees observing. The staff provided additional information regarding psychological testing and a treatment course. Then there was a lively discussion about diagnosis. One of the senior staff voiced the same sentiment I had heard more than thirty years earlier: "Don't use the word *schizophrenia* yet. Let's wait."

This book counters the assumptions that underlie those statements: that using the word *schizophrenia* should be shunned for as long as possible; that using it as the diagnosis of a patient is necessarily a bad thing; and that people for whom it is an appropriate diagnosis have no hope and no expectations.

Diagnosis: Schizophrenia was written by Rachel Miller, L.C.S.W., Ph.D., Susan Mason, Ph.D., and a group of patients who participated in the New Onset Psychosis Program at The Zucker Hillside Hospital, a division of North Shore–Long Island Jewish Health System. It grew out of the patients' desire to share with others their experiences with the illness and how they have coped with and solved problems. The initial experience of schizophrenia can be frightening, and the chapters that follow, told by people "who have been there," are designed to help chart a path toward recovery.

We hope that *Diagnosis: Schizophrenia* will find a place in hospital waiting rooms, in social workers' offices, and in the back pockets of patients and their families who have just heard the diagnosis of schizophrenia for the first time. Its purpose is to develop and strengthen understanding and offer tools for patients, their families, and those who provide treatment. The chapters are short and to the point, and they cover a wide range of issues from hospitalization to rehabilitation. Dip in and read a chapter that deals with a current problem, or read the book cover to cover. *Diagnosis: Schizophrenia* brings a new perspective to the information on coping with mental illness that is available through a range of sources.

Nina Schooler, Ph.D.
Director of Research
Hillside Hospital
North Shore–Long Island Jewish Health System

Introductory Note

Eight years after the first edition of *Diagnosis: Schizophrenia*'s publication, much has changed and little has changed. New medications have been developed and our understanding of schizophrenia has expanded. Yet, young people continue to develop schizophrenia, with the same symptoms and the same struggles with recovery as the thirty-five people in this book share.

When we—thirty-five young people newly diagnosed with schizophrenia plus two social workers—embarked on the four-year journey of planning, interviewing, illustrating, reviewing, editing, and finding a publisher for the first edition, we had little idea of the difficulty we would have interesting a publisher in a book that primarily was written for people with schizophrenia. Fortunately, we found John Michel of Columbia University Press, who saw the promise of this book. Now, thousands of copies later and with feedback from many young people who were helped by it, the stigma is just a little bit lessened. When we began, there were no other books targeted to people with schizophrenia; now we are happy to say there are several.

The purpose of this book, back in 2002 and now, is to tell the story of thirty-five young people coping with an illness that completely upended their lives. In so doing, we all hope to help others with schizophrenia, as well as anyone else who might benefit from better understanding the issues of recovering from the disease. Initially we thought the book would be about their stories, but by the second brainstorming session we quickly learned that people wanted to know everything, all the science, about the medications, how the doctors decide it is schizophrenia, even what the therapists were doing to help and why. As the editors we respected their concerns and included a great deal more than originally planned. In that spirit, in this edition we have expanded numerous sections to provide recent scientific findings, updates of benefit information, additional material for coping with symptoms, issues of substance abuse treatment, and information regarding childhood-onset schizophrenia. We have added many new resources available via the Internet and print materials. As with the first edition, we did our best to make the book as readable as possible, taking into consideration the difficulties in concentration sometimes experienced by people with schizophrenia.

Where we have made no changes is to the stories of the thirty-five people who so courageously shared their most difficult experiences with us. Unfortunately, we no longer have contact with the participants who were so important to this project. Many kept in touch with Rachel Miller until her move to Maryland. One person, who was very involved in this book, stopped her medication after many years and numerous personal successes and took a while to recover again. Another told the story of how her doctor recommended she read *Diagnosis: Schizophrenia*. She replied proudly, "I'm one of the people in it." When the doctor asked, "Which one?" she responded that this was her secret. One young man found Rachel Miller at her new job at the National Institute of Mental Health last year to ask a question about anxiety; another to get help for a brother. Several people participated in radio programs to promote the book in which they spoke of their experiences. We hope all thirty-five young people continue to progress in their recoveries. If any one of you is reading this, please know that we continue to hear from people around the world about how this book you helped to outline, gave your voice, illustrated, edited, and finally celebrated (remember our party) continues to live in a second edition. More than that, your hopefulness and work toward recovery tell the world that young people newly diagnosed who have good treatment can optimize their recoveries and lead meaningful lives. We know we can speak for you when we say it is our hope that the second edition of this book will make the journey for people recently diagnosed with schizophrenia a little bit easier.

We profoundly thank our participants for their help in enlightening us in ways no one else possibly could. In addition, we wish to thank all the research doctors and other professionals who contributed their knowledge to *Diagnosis: Schizophrenia*. We also are very grateful to the Nicholas Family Charitable Trust, which provided generous support for this project.

Rachel Miller, Bethesda, Maryland

Susan E. Mason, New York City, New York

A Note on the Title

Schizophrenia is a complex illness with several subtypes, as described on pages 57 to 59. Schizoaffective disorder is a closely related disorder and is often described as schizophrenia with significant mood symptoms (see pages 60 to 61). In *Diagnosis: Schizophrenia*, we refer to both disorders as "schizophrenia," although several of the thirty-five participants were diagnosed with schizoaffective disorder. In this way we hope to simplify the book. Most important, the issues and treatment for schizophrenia and schizoaffective disorder are very similar.

Acknowledgments

We would like to thank a number of people for their support and help in making this book possible. First, we would like to give special recognition to all the young people who participated by providing their ideas for the book as well as their individual stories. In addition, we wish to acknowledge all the participants with schizophrenia who worked with us to "test" the book during the editing process. We thank John M. Kane, M.D., Chairman of the Department of Psychiatry for North Shore–Long Island Jewish Health System, for his support of our work within the hospital and research setting. To our colleagues at Zucker Hillside Hospital Research Center we owe our gratitude for their unending support and willingness to contribute significant sections whenever called upon. Joanne McCormack, M.S.W., continues to be an enormous help in keeping our project going at Zucker Hillside Hospital, sharing our book with people around the United States, and helping with diagnostic updates. Brian Sheitman, M.D., whose respect and caring for young people with schizophrenia was inspiring, also provided important seeds of encouragement early in planning. For the graphics of Low III, a self-stigmatizing female, and sketches of individual participants, we wish to acknowledge Audrey and Zelda, whose true names we are unable to provide. For the graphics of the brain and neurons, we wish to thank Handan Gunduz-Bruce, M.D.

The Nicholas Family Charitable Trust made it possible to fund this project, and Lynn Nicholas, Ph.D., in particular, offered faith in our endeavor throughout its four-year undertaking. We also wish to acknowledge our previous editor, John Michel, for his confidence in our project and commitment to bringing the first edition of this book to fruition. His death on January 30, 2005, was a great loss for us, though we continue to be inspired by his good nature and fine mind. We wish to thank our current editor, Lauren Dockett, who carries on in the tradition of John Michel and provided guidance as we updated *Diagnosis: Schizophrenia* to reflect advances in understanding and treatment of schizophrenia. At the National Institute of Mental Health, Judith Rapoport, M.D., has been exceptionally supportive of the addition of childhood-onset schizophrenia to the new edition. Together with Dr. Rapoport, Julia Tossell, M.D., and Nitin Gogtay, M.D., provided the mentoring necessary for understanding childhood schizophrenia. At Yeshiva University's Wurzweiler School of Social Work, thanks to our colleagues, who gave us encouragement and support, especially Dean Sheldon Gelman and Yeshiva University Provost Morton Lowengrub for their continued support. Also at Yeshiva, Zalmon Rothchild, M.A., provided invaluable research assistance for this second edition. Richard A. Schere, Ph.D., who was kind enough to read the first draft, provided comments that helped us to make the book more accessible to readers. For his legal assistance we wish to thank Victor Serby, J.D. Last but not least, we wish to thank Walter Miller for his patience and loving understanding of the importance of this project and grandsons Daniel and Mark Hooks for the nourishment of their hugs and kisses.

Rachel Miller receives no income from the publication of *Diagnosis: Schizophrenia.*

Susan Mason has designated 50 percent of proceeds from *Diagnosis: Schizophrenia* to schizophrenia research at Zucker Hillside Hospital.

The views of the authors do not necessarily represent the views of the NIH.

About the Authors

Participant-Authors. All the participant-authors took part in a National Institute of Mental Health research project at Zucker Hillside Hospital, North Shore–Long Island Jewish Health System, to further the understanding of the first episode of schizophrenia. Their ages ranged from seventeen to thirty-nine. Some were in high school or college, while others had completed college or were working at the time of their first hospitalization. They were from many backgrounds, including Irish, Italian, Haitian, Puerto Rican, African American, Jewish, German, Polish, Russian, Chinese, Korean, Filipino, Indian, Guyanese, and Jamaican.

Stephen Anderson, M.A. received his master's in rehabilitation counseling from New York University. For thirty years he worked at Fountain House, a nonprofit organization in New York City. His contributions there were numerous, including developing programs for independent employment, education, and training on the principles of clubhouse models. He served on the faculty of the International Center for Clubhouse Development, where he also provided consulting services and certification. Mr. Anderson contributes to us his knowledge of the clubhouse.

Julia Becker, M.D. is currently assistant professor of psychiatry at Weill Cornell Medical College and is an attending psychiatrist at New York Presbyterian Hospital, White Plains, New York. She has a private practice in Forest Hills, New York. She received her Doctor of Medicine degree from the Indiana University School of Medicine, Bloomington, and her postgraduate training at the University of Chicago and Zucker

Hillside Hospital. She is the recipient of several awards, including the International Congress of Schizophrenia Young Investigator Award. She is Board certified in psychiatry, neurology, and forensic psychiatry. Dr. Becker's work at Zucker Hillside Hospital included teaching, supervising, and lecturing medical students and residents. She also served as Medical Director of the RAP (Recognition and Prevention of Psychological Problems) Clinic and as an attending psychiatrist in the Zucker Hillside Hospital Research Department. Her research work and publications are in the areas of first-episode schizophrenia, schizophrenia, schizoaffective disorder, early intervention studies, obsessive-compulsive disorder, mania and depression, and psychopharmacology.

Handan Gunduz-Bruce, M.D. received her Doctor of Medicine degree from the University of Istanbul and her postgraduate training at the University of Istanbul, New York Medical College, and Zucker Hillside Hospital of the Albert Einstein College of Medicine. She is currently an attending psychiatrist in the Department of Psychiatry of Yale Medical School and the West Haven VA, and principal investigator of several studies researching the pathogenesis of schizophrenia using imaging and electrophysiological tools. During her tenure at Zucker Hillside Hospital, she served as the medical coordinator of the Neuroimaging Unit of the Mental Health Clinic Research Center and was also involved with several additional research studies, including the First Episode of Schizophrenia Studies.

Anil Malhotra, M.D. is Director of Psychiatry Research at the Zucker Hillside Hospital in Glen Oaks, New York and Associate Professor of Psychiatry at the Albert Einstein College of Medicine (AECOM) in the Bronx, New York. Dr. Malhotra completed his undergraduate studies at Cornell University in 1985 and received his M.D. from Wake Forest University in 1989. After residency training in psychiatry at Georgetown University, he completed a research fellowship at the National Institute of Mental Health (NIMH) of the National Institutes of Health (NIH).

Dr. Malhotra developed a research program in pharmacogenetics at the NIMH and was appointed the Chief of the Unit of Pharmacogenetics in the Experimental Therapeutics Branch in 1996. In 1998, Dr. Malhotra moved to the Zucker Hillside Hospital and AECOM to develop a molecular genetics program focused on the major neuropsychiatric disorders. Dr. Malhotra's current research interests are the role of molecular factors in human cognition and the pharmacogenetics of antipsychotic drug response. He has conducted a series of studies implicating the glutamatergic N-methyl-d-aspartate (NMDA) receptor in neurocognition, as well as molecular studies identifying key candidate genes for specific aspects of human cognition. His work in pharmacogenetics has primarily focused on variation in the neurotransmitter receptor genes and their relationship to clinical response to the atypical antipsychotic agent, clozapine. Dr. Malhotra has published more than seventy peer-reviewed papers in these areas as well as numerous review articles and book chapters. Dr. Malhotra receives grant support from the NIH, philanthropic foundations including the Stanley Foundation and the National Alliance for Research in Schizophrenia and Affective Disorders (NARSAD), and private industry.

Susanne Mars, C.R.C., L.M.H.C. received a master's degree from New York University before beginning a long tenure with the Psychiatric Rehabilitation Department at Zucker Hillside Hospital. She began her work as a rehabilitation counselor with adults on inpatient units and in ambulatory care. She trained and supervised psychiatric rehabilitation staff and students and developed rehabilitation programs for all inpatient units, including specialty units such as first-episode schizophrenia, mentally ill chemical abusers, mentally retarded dual diagnosis, and dialectical behavioral treatment. She recently terminated her position at Zucker Hillside Hospital as manager of Psychiatric Rehabilitation Services and devotes her professional time to her private practice in counseling and psychotherapy in Lakewood, New Jersey. Her credentials include licenses in mental health counseling (New York), professional counseling (New Jersey), and rehabilitation counseling (New Jersey). She recently completed advanced training in modern psychoanalysis at the Center for Modern Psychoanalytic Studies in New York City. She has also written about psychiatric rehabilitation programming for polysubstance abuse treatment.

Susan E. Mason, M.S.S.W., Ph.D. graduated from the Columbia School of Social Work. She holds several additional degrees, including a Ph.D. in sociology and education from Columbia University, a master's in health administration from New York University, and a certificate in psychoanalytic psychotherapy from the Washington Square Institute in New York City. Dr. Mason worked with people diagnosed with schizophrenia at Jacobi, Mount Sinai, and Zucker Hillside Hospitals. At Zucker Hillside Hospital she managed several clinical trials for psychotropic medications for schizophrenia. She is currently professor of social work at Wurzweiler School of Social Work, Yeshiva University and professor of sociology for the university's college programs. She is the author of more than forty peer-reviewed journal articles, seven of which are coauthored with Rachel Miller on schizophrenia treatment. Dr. Mason is coeditor of *Community Health Care in Cuba* (2009), in which she has written chapters on mental health care for both adolescents and adults and on HIV interventions. She continues to conduct research and write extensively on the treatment of schizophrenia and other psychiatric disorders.

Alan Mendelowitz, M.D. received his Doctor of Medicine degree from Rutgers Medical School, Piscataway, New Jersey, and his postgraduate training at Hillside Hospital. He has been adjunct professor in the Hunter College masters' program in rehabilitation counseling and consulting psychiatrist for the Epilepsy Center at Long Island Jewish Medical Center. He is currently the Unit Chief of Low III at Hillside Hospital, with responsibility for residency training. In addition, he is an associate professor of psychiatry at Albert Einstein College of Medicine, Bronx, New York. Dr. Mendelowitz's research interests center on relapse prevention in schizophrenia. His publications focus on antipsychotic and antidepressant medications, side effects, and schizophrenia. Dr. Mendelowitz has been honored as one of *New York* Magazine's "Top Doctors in New York" and Castle Connolly's "Top Physicians in the North East."

Rachel Miller, M.S.W, Ph.D. earned her Master of Social Work degree and Ph.D. from Adelphi School of Social Work, Garden City, New York and a certificate in psychoanalytic psychotherapy from the New York School for Psychoanalytic Psychotherapy and Psychoanalysis. She has extensive experience working with young people with schizophrenia, especially those experiencing the first episode of illness. Dr. Miller is a licensed clinical social worker who worked in inpatient and outpatient treatment for the Research Department of Zucker Hillside Hospital's Continuous Care Team for first-episode patients for twelve years. Currently she is a research social worker at the National Institute of Mental Health (NIMH), Child Psychiatry Branch, where her work is focused on childhood-onset schizophrenia. She is a consultant for Recovery After an Initial Schizophrenia Episode (RAISE), a large NIMH initiative to improve long-term outcomes. She has published and presented in the areas of phase-specific treatment, group modality, adherence to treatment, cannabis use, cognitive enhancement, integrated treatment, shame and guilt, faith and spirituality, and prevention of HIV, all as related to first-episode schizophrenia. Dr. Miller has been on the editorial board of *SZ Magazine*, previously *Schizophrenia Digest*, since 2003. She has consulted for pharmaceutical companies to provide consumer education materials. Prior to her career in social work, Dr. Miller worked as an educational writer.

Linda Porto, M.S.N., R.N.C.S., N.P.P. is a licensed nurse practitioner and registered professional nurse. She received her M.S.N. from Adelphi University, Garden City, New York and has a certificate in holistic nursing from New York College for Holistic Health, Education and Research. Over the years she provided psychiatric nursing services to adults and adolescents in inpatient and outpatient settings. Ms. Porto worked as a clinical interviewer and research nurse in the Department of Psychiatry Research at Zucker Hillside Hospital. Currently she is a psychiatric nurse practitioner at Family Continuity Inc. in Hyannis, Massachusetts, where she works with children, adolescents, and adults. Through her agency's contract with the Massachusetts Department of Youth Services, she helps young people with substance abuse and mental health issues. She has co-authored several articles on schizophrenia and co-occurring syndromes.

Delbert G. Robinson, M.D. is a professor of psychiatry and behavioral sciences at the Albert Einstein College of Medicine. He has been the principal investigator of National Institute of Mental Health–funded studies of the treatment of first-episode schizophrenia and also of methods to enhance antipsychotic medication adherence. His first-episode schizophrenia research has focused upon first-episode treatment response, relapse prevention, and recovery. He is one of the leading authorities on the pharmacotherapy for first-episode illness. He was a member of the Psychopharmacologic Drugs Advisory Committee of the Food and Drug Administration from 2004 to 2008. In 2000 Dr. Robinson received the Exemplary Psychiatrists Award from the National Alliance for the Mentally Ill.

Nina R. Schooler, Ph.D., professor of psychiatry and behavioral sciences at the State University of New York in Brooklyn, New York, earned her doctorate in social psychology from Columbia University. A former member of the Psychopharmacologic Drug Advisory Committee of the Food and Drug Administration, Dr. Schooler currently chairs one of the

NIMH Data Safety Monitoring Boards and has served NIMH as a consultant in many other capacities. She was president of the Association for Clinical Psychosocial Research and the American Psychopathological Association, as well as a fellow of the American Psychological Association and the American College of Neuropsychopharmacology. Dr. Schooler has received the Gralnick Foundation High Point Hospital Award from the National Association of Health Services, the Alexander Gralnick Award from the American Psychological Foundation, and the Hogarty Excellence in Schizophrenia Award from the University of Pittsburgh. In addition to contributing to a number of textbook chapters on the evaluation of pharmacological treatments of schizophrenia, she has published her research findings on maintenance treatment, relapse, and rehospitalization and treatment of first-episode schizophrenia in academic journals.

Mary L. Trump, Ph.D., has a master's in English literature from Columbia University, New York, and a master's and Ph.D in psychology from Adelphi University, Garden City, New York. Ms. Trump worked closely with Rachel Miller during the preparation of the first edition of *Diagnosis: Schizophrenia*.

Research assistance was provided by **Zalman Rothchild, M.A.** He has a B.A. from Binghamton University, Binghamton, New York and an M.A. from Yeshiva University, New York, New York.

Using This Book

- Feel free to skip around. You can read as much or as little as you like. If you have trouble concentrating, read very small sections, then stop. In time you will be able to read more easily.
- Encourage your family members and friends to read this book. It will help them to understand what you are going through.
- Chapters 1 through 15 contain several personal stories. They are real stories, but we are not using the real names of people, schools, or towns. If you are curious to find out how the people in these stories are doing, turn to chapter 15 at any time.
- There are several sections providing information about medication, social services, and rehabilitation services. You may use these sections as reference tools when you need specific information, but this book does not replace your doctor and therapist. It is simply another resource for you and your family.
- Some of the medical information is very technical. Do not get upset if you don't understand it fully. It is very difficult. In fact, only people with many years of training can really comprehend the details, and even the experts don't understand everything about how the brain or medicines work. Look for the brief, easier explanations of the more difficult material.
- If you have questions, write them down in the margins. Then you can get answers from your doctor, therapist, or even NAMI (National Association of the Mentally Ill).

- Unfortunately, Web sites sometimes change. If a URL we provide does not work, try to find the organization mentioned by searching the Web.
- Remember, every one of the people whose stories you will read is rooting for you.

This book does not replace your doctor and therapist.

DIAGNOSIS: SCHIZOPHRENIA

INTRODUCTION

So They Say We Have Schizophrenia

All illnesses are hard to talk about, but schizophrenia seems even harder. For many people the term carries a stigma so strong that just thinking about it is frightening. It reminds them of the strange thoughts, feelings, and behaviors that resulted in their needing treatment. They remember their weird beliefs and hallucinations or their disorganized, isolated, or moody ways.

Once the symptoms of schizophrenia improve, people want to put the terrifying events of their illness and treatment behind them. They want to forget. Yet, like all other serious illnesses, schizophrenia needs to be talked about. If people do not talk about their experiences with this disease, they will not learn from them and will have little control over what happens to them.

A couple of years ago, during one of our group therapy sessions, we were discussing how much had changed for us.

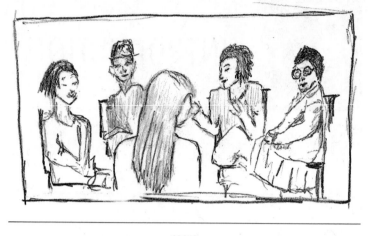

GROUP

Here's what happened.

JOSEPH: It's hard for me to believe now, but I really thought the FBI was after me.

AMBER: You too? I thought every time I went to the bathroom there was a camera in the ceiling where they watched me. I wouldn't tell anyone, but I was so scared I wouldn't go to the bathroom. I wasn't telling them a thing.

MEREDITH: I know about that. One day I was sitting in the chair in my room. The sun was pouring in over my shoulder, shining on me. And I was sure I was the Virgin Mary. The doctor asked me, "Do you feel there is anything special about you?" I looked him straight in the eye and said, "Nope."

JOSEPH: They would ask me questions. Did I think someone wanted to hurt me? No way I was going to tell them. I thought they were all in on the plot. You know that Dr. Mendelowitz? I thought he was the head of the Mafia.

MEREDITH: Him? Wow!

RACHEL (social worker): I remember how frightening that was for you then, but today you're all laughing.

JOSEPH: Well, it's funny when you think about it now. You need to be able to laugh about it.

MEREDITH: And you can't do that with other people.

AMBER: They wouldn't understand.

RACHEL: What about people who don't know anyone else who has this illness? What could we do to help them be able to laugh and not feel so alone?

AMBER: You mean something like our poem?

MEREDITH: That's an idea. We could write something.

RACHEL: How about a book? Would you be interested in doing something like that?

JOSEPH: Wow! That sounds good.

AMBER: Do you think we could do it?

RACHEL: Let me set up some meetings to see if other people might want to write a book.

That's how this project started. And yes, we did want to write a book. We hope you won't be afraid to share the story of our journey.

So they say we have schizophrenia. Well, when they first told most of us we didn't believe it, or want to believe it. But it's been a while, and now we understand it, as much as anyone can. Having been through it, we would like to share our experiences with other people for a lot of reasons.

- We don't want people who get ill to feel so alone.
- The experience was so scary, and we think knowing what to expect might make it less scary.
- We want to change the negative stereotypes people associate with schizophrenia.
- We want to explain that the symptoms are part of the illness—they have nothing to do with the kind of person who has the illness.
- We want to show that people with schizophrenia do get better—there is hope.
- We want to show that having schizophrenia does not mean you will hurt other people.
- So many people have helped us; we want to do our part to help others.

This is our story. We hope it helps.

Abby	Buddy	Linda	Sam
Alexandra	Gary	Lucinda	Samantha

Alexis	Genevive	Marcus	Sasha
Amber	Ilan	Mark	Sharon
Audrey	Jackie	Meredith	Smokey
Beaux	James	Mike	Thomas
Ben	Jeff	Patrick	Van
Beth	Joseph	Richie	Vanessa
Buck	Laurie	Roman	Zelda

4

We have been studying the first episode of schizophrenia at our research center for nearly thirty years, and we have learned a lot. Much of what we have learned is included in this book. We could never have done this research without the help of the young people in our program.

Rachel Miller, L.C.S.W, Ph.D.
Susan E. Mason, L.C.S.W., Ph.D.
Julia Becker, M.D.
Handan Gunduz-Bruce, M.D.
Anil Malhotra, M.D.
Susanne Mars, C.R.C., C.C.M.H.
Joanne McCormack, C.S.W.
Alan Mendelowitz, M.D.
Linda Porto, R.N.
Delbert Robinson, M.D.

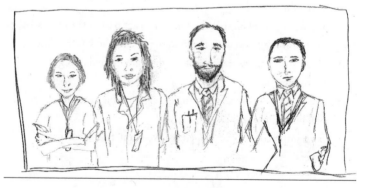

STAFF

North Shore–Long Island Jewish Health System
Zucker Hillside Hospital Research Center

1 IN THE BEGINNING

For some of us, schizophrenia came on suddenly and turned our lives inside out overnight. Others became ill over a long period of time, so our lives took a slow downward turn. In both cases, treating the symptoms of schizophrenia required hospitalization to keep us safe until our symptoms were under control. It allowed staff to provide treatment in a more complete way: the medication was adjusted to the right level and any reactions were carefully checked and treated. We also had the opportunity to learn more about caring for ourselves. Despite these advantages, we know the hospital experience can be very hard and frightening. We hope that hearing some of our stories will make you feel less alone.

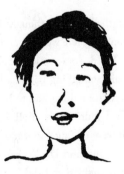

GENEVIVE

GENEVIVE: I was twenty-four and was working as a home health aide. While I was working I started to have symptoms. I thought people were after me and I was being followed. I thought my phone was tapped. The office would call me to tell me where I was going to be working. The ones spying on me were people I didn't know, but I gave them names. I went to the office to quit because I thought people were following me. I stayed home and I got worse. I thought my house was bugged. I thought those people knew what I was wearing and what I was doing. I thought they were going to defame me on TV. I thought they put a camera in my house. One day I cut a wire and my father got upset. I had my brother search the whole house. The voices told me it was this tiny little camera.

I was hearing voices saying they were going to kill my father, rape me, kill me. I stopped eating to end this, to die. I didn't trust anyone. I thought there was this FBI agent, one of the neighbors, who was going to protect me. When I asked my mother why she was trying to poison me, she would get upset with me. That confirmed my belief she was trying to poison me. Really she wasn't doing that, but that's what I felt. I didn't even know I was sick until I came to the hospital and Dr. Gunduz started questioning me. That's when I knew.

When I was in my room there was a car parked outside that I could see from my window on Low III, an inpatient unit at Zucker Hillside Hospital. I thought it was an FBI agent there to protect me. I thought he was saying that he wanted me to have the best room. Then when they moved me to a better room I thought, wow, he was my advocate and he got me this really good room. I remember that I started to feel better when I was given medication.

At first when I was in the hospital I thought I wouldn't be in for long. I thought there were people in there worse than I was. It was like a prison really. That's how I felt. The doors were locked. I felt trapped. I was put in this place because I did something bad. I asked this girl, "What are you in for?" You had to do something bad to be in a mental institution. I remember my first day. I didn't sleep at all. I sat on the dining room chair. I thought the staff were talking about me. Then on the second day I met Ms. Miller, Dr. Gunduz, and Dr. Becker. I didn't know what was happening to me. I just thought that I did something bad to my niece and nephew. It was not until I got out of the hospital that my sister and mother told me I didn't do anything bad at all. It was the illness that caused me to think that.

JAMES: I was twenty-two three years ago. I was confused. I didn't know what was going on. I thought my grandmother and my grandfather were trying to drug me with food. I always knew the feeling of being confused, but this was heightened. I was doing things I wouldn't normally do, like I would be off sometimes by an hour when I was telling time. I was starting to hear things and I would think that other people were talking about me. I would think that people were reading my mind, but really it was just the sickness. One other symptom I had was I used to get a lot of headaches and I was thirsty all the time. There were a lot of symptoms that scared me. At the time I was going through a divorce also. I thought it was all one big joke.

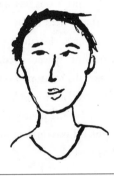

JAMES

When I came to the hospital I thought I was going to pass this test and I would be with my wife again. When I finally came out I realized that it wasn't a big game. Also, after a couple of weeks I knew that it was serious. When I first went in there they had me in a room, isolated, trying different drugs. Then one of the orderlies asked another patient to show me around. I guess when you are in the hospital you find your help from people that are in the hospital with you. Don't let the screaming patients scare you. Don't let the restraints scare you. They are there for your safety.

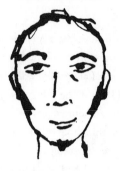

ROMAN

ROMAN: I was twenty-six and working at a bank. I thought people were after me, people wanted to kill me. I was hearing voices. I took off from where I was living with a girl and went to my father's. I got five minutes of peace and then started hearing voices, cursing me out, saying they were going to kill me. I really thought they were outside. They were so audible. I thought there were snipers on the rooftops. I was hiding behind the wall in the kitchen. I thought they had ultraviolet laser vision. I told my father to call the police for help. I called the police three times. The third time the cop asked if I was all right, if I was on anything.

It was scary being in the hospital.

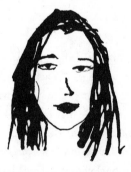

JACKIE

JACKIE: They brought me to the hospital and I thought they were dropping me off and leaving me there for good. I sat in the chair, and the nurse was going through my bags for anything sharp to take away. I was looking at the people and started shaking. I was really scared. They finished and put me in a room with a very nice girl with whom I became friends. The next day I saw about five or six doctors at one time and they all were asking me about my experience. The voices in my head were telling me when to say yes and when to say no and when not to say anything. They put me on Prolixin the next day. I don't know how long it took to get better, but I was in the hospital for six weeks. I made a lot of friends. We played games and talked. We just got better together.

SHARON: It all started one snowy day away at school when I was nineteen. I did a flip on my bed. I don't remember clearly, but it was like a dream. They told me if I didn't get help they were going to terminate me from school. I went to the hospital looking real weird. My hair was sticking up on top of my head, and I wasn't in my right mind. They tried to get me to eat, but I just picked at my food. I was very afraid and scared. The next thing I knew I woke up strapped down to a bed. When I looked up I saw my mother. I smiled at her. I couldn't touch her. I couldn't hold her. I couldn't kiss her. But I knew she was my mother. People told her not to come up in all the snow because I wouldn't know her, but she did.

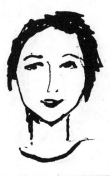

SHARON

I went home with my mother for a few weeks. The second day home I couldn't walk and I was foaming from the mouth. My mother took me to a local hospital and [the doctors] told her that the hospital upstate had given me an overdose of medication. They gave me the right dosage of Haldol and I was able to go home to my mother's house. When I got home I was very afraid to come out of my room. I would get up in the morning, take a bath, and just go back to my room and lie in bed. I packed all my clothes because I thought I was going away somewhere. Then on certain days I would strip naked and climb into the closet like I was in prison in the Middle East. One day my little brother came down and he saw me. He asked my mother, "Why is Sharon downstairs naked in the closet?" I was very paranoid. I was scared that people were going to kill me. I thought there were helicopters flying over my house with people who knew about all the bad things I did in my life. They were going to kill me. I saw men on the wall and I saw visions of guns pointing in my direction. It was very, very scary. It was amazing that I lived from one day to the next with the constant fear.

Finally my mother got me some help and I started seeing this doctor. I told her what was going on and she finally admitted me to Zucker Hillside Hospital. I was put in Zucker Hillside on Low III. I hated being locked up with nowhere to go. Because of the state I was in, I gave the staff a lot of trouble, so I was getting injectable medication to keep me calm. I wouldn't take the other medication. I just never liked it. When I went to group, I learned a lot about my illness, and I started taking my medicine regularly. I got better.

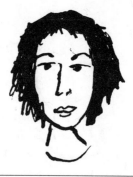

MEREDITH

MEREDITH: Three years ago I started becoming very emotional and crying a lot. I would cry often; I'd also feel high and very happy. I always thought that was the way I was naturally, but it was to the extreme. I started having strange thoughts, like the end of the world was coming. I started feeling things like heartbeats in my stomach, and I thought I was pregnant with Jesus Christ. I thought I was crazy. One day I woke up at 5 a.m. and I went down to where my mom and dad sleep. I woke my dad. We were talking and suddenly I had the fear he was the devil. It scared me so that I ran up to the attic. I kept trying to get my sister to jump out the window. My dad ran after me. When I saw him I stuck my leg out the window. My sister pulled me back in. All I could scream was "God" because I was so afraid. We all went to church and talked to the priest after the mass. I told him I was going to have Jesus Christ, and he told my parents to bring me to the hospital.

11

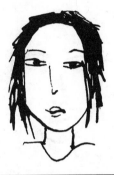

ABBY

ABBY: I'm twenty-eight years old. I was born October 12. I have four sisters and three brothers. I was working in a large department store as a customer service representative. I wrote a rap song around the time I got sick and I was hoping to get my music started. I was twenty-four years old when I got sick. I was going through some problems with the people that lived in my neighborhood. I don't think I was comfortable living there. I thought some people didn't like me; maybe it was jealousy. I just started feeling worried about things. Then I went to a religious store and I was trying to let this man in the store know how I felt. I kept going back to the store when something was bothering me. I went to a psychiatrist and let him know how I felt. I was trying to get help because my emotions were being controlled and my thoughts were being controlled. Sometimes it even felt like my movements were being controlled. And I was very uncomfortable.

The first time I was admitted in the hospital I was comfortable because I think I needed to be calmed down. I felt like I needed to get away to try to put things together. There were two little incidents when I was in the hospital that I remember. One man came in and kicked my bed to wake me up. One lady went to draw my blood. I was trying to explain something about drawing my blood and she grabbed my arm, trying to tell me I had to get my blood drawn. I wasn't used to getting my blood drawn so many times. I wasn't used to the routine. My mother had a stroke when I was in the hospital. I was frightened because when I was talking to her over the phone she wasn't talking right. That scared me and I wanted to leave the hospital to see my mother.

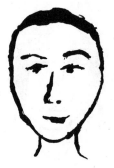

JEFF

JEFF: Two years ago I was having some problems with my next-door neighbors. They were making accusations, fighting with my father, and taking parts off my car. I really wanted to get back at them because I was getting really tired of it. I went out to get a permit for a gun, but it was too much trouble to have a gun. Mainly I was having problems with the neighbors talking about me. I talked with my mother, but that wasn't enough to get rid of these problems.

I was on Low III for three weeks and then I was in day hospital for two or three months. Then I got jobs. I am a car mechanic, so the first one was at a tire shop and the next was at a transmission shop. For the last year I've been working at a transmission shop, and that's pretty much where I am now.

It was not fun being in the hospital. I got conjunctivitis. The first night, I was robbed of all my money. I got jock itch. Other than that, it was okay. I got through it.

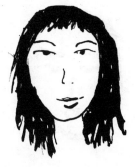

ALEXANDRA

ALEXANDRA: I was in the hospital in January four years ago. I was diagnosed with schizophrenia. I was hearing voices. They were like voices coming from the vent in my room. I couldn't get the voices out of my head. I think that they were saying things in the basement. I don't remember anymore. It's still frightening to talk about it. I didn't know I was going to go into the hospital that day. I didn't want to stay, but they told me I had to stay, and it took me a long time to get out. I missed my cousin's wedding that year. I didn't like that at all. They were giving me too much medicine. I hated getting up at 7 a.m. to get my meds and breakfast. I was so tired from the medicine. They had these groups I didn't want to go to because I was so tired all the time. They had awful lunches.

I was in the hospital a couple of times. All I wanted was to go home. I kept calling my parents every day, every hour. I think I was there for months. I wanted to go home so badly.

I was so scared of staying in that place. They would wake you up with the light, every hour on the hour. They put the flashlight in the room to see if we were breathing.

I kept asking the doctor, "When am I going home?"

"Why did I have to come to the hospital?"

"Why do I have to stay so long?"

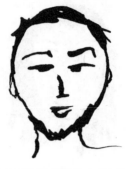

THOMAS

THOMAS: I came to the hospital because I was having panic attacks. I was very disoriented. I was starting to feel closed in the house. I started to get very depressed. I felt like people were looking at me strangely and saying things about me. It was okay in the hospital. I just needed some time away from my house. I came to the hospital. I wanted to be there but I didn't at the same time. I knew I needed help but I wanted to be at home. I think the hospital helped me.

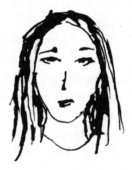

VANESSA

VANESSA: When I was about thirty-five years old my illness started. I couldn't get out of bed. I was crying a lot. I tried to turn on the TV to relax me and I would hear the voices. I would change the channel on the TV and more voices. So I cut the TV off. I tried to do the laundry, started crying, and couldn't finish the laundry. I heard voices in my head. They were the voices of friends, family members. I sat on the couch and started crying again. I got up, got dressed, dressed my two children, and went to my mother's house. I started crying over there and tried to explain to her what was going on. I told her to call the ambulance. The police came. The ambulance came. They questioned me for a little while. Then they took me to Queens General. My mother and father followed in the car with my children. From there they transferred me to Zucker Hillside Hospital.

The hospital was scary. I couldn't sleep all night. They put me in a room by myself. The mattress was on the floor. I kept hearing voices. I got up a couple of times while I was in the room. I got up and asked the nurse to give me something to help me sleep. The next morning they put me in a room with another girl. We talked for a little while and I found out that she had similar symptoms to mine. Later the doctor came in. He spoke to me, questioned me. Then he prescribed my medication for me.

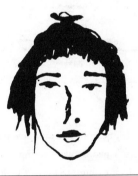

SAM

SAM: I have been 9,000 miles away before, but I never felt so isolated as when I was in the hospital. I felt fear. I used to call home at least five times a day. I would ask my mom to take me home. The first couple of days, everyone came to visit me. My sister-in-law came to visit, but I don't recall. My mind became numb. It was like when your finger freezes and you hit it: I was totally oblivious for the first week. I saw strange faces; I remember a guy who shaved half his face and he was very skinny. One time he had a fight and four security guards couldn't hold him down. I became so scared. In addition to being sick, I had an unreasonable fear. I was there for six weeks. You can get used to anything. I fell into the routine; I wasn't as anxious to get out.

BEAUX: It all began when I was twenty-six. I started to read a self-help book and I was getting deeply into it, like brainwashed. I had been a smoker for quite a few years but I gave that up cold turkey. Then within a couple of days I started getting visions. I saw people who were dead and then I just felt total confusion. By then I realized I had a problem, and I was afraid. I had a car accident and came into the hospital. At first my family didn't want to admit me. I didn't want to be admitted either. The next thing I realized I was on Low III. It was kind of intimidating, because you know there's something wrong but you can't control it.

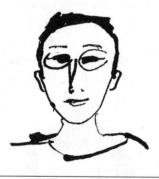

BEAUX

I think it was tough to try to heal around everybody else who had the same set of problems. I felt people were acting strange, including myself. When you have delusions it's tough to know the difference between what is real and what is not. For example, I was eating a meal and somebody jumped up behind me and sat right back down. It doesn't seem like much, but when you're in there it adds to the confusion. That was the toughest part.

SAMANTHA: I was hospitalized for two months on Low III. In addition to being in a locked unit, they have this policy of status on Low III. You had to follow all their procedures. You start out with no privileges at all. You eat on the unit. You're not allowed to go home. You're not allowed to go out. At first I was uncooperative and I didn't wish to take medication. Different doctors talked to me about my symptoms and starting medication. I was unhappy with my living situation. I would stand at the window and scream for no reason. I was paranoid. I thought there was a man bothering me, which was probably part of my illness. I just felt he was there to bother me. But in time I gave in, cooperated, took my medication, participated in the activities, and slowly I earned my way up the status ladder.

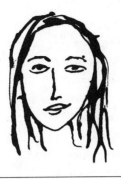

SAMANTHA

At one time I had a misunderstanding with one of the staff. She had lied to me about something and I was so upset to find out she had lied. I took this deck of cards and threw them at her. Six aides came and took me into a room that was empty except for a mattress on the floor. I went to sleep on the mat for three hours. When I woke up I sort of cried a little bit. They came back at lunchtime and let me out. So I had an example of what happens when you have an outburst like that. There were other people who had outbursts and they would restrain them to the bed, and they couldn't get up at all; they had to have a round-the-clock person sitting there all the time. Once I cooperated with the rules, took my medication, and followed their routine, I was permitted more and more privileges.

This poem was written by one of our group and has been helpful to us all as we've come to understand the experience of being in the hospital.

THE HOSPITAL

Blank walls suspended in space
Fearful faces, what is this place?
Stale food, locked by doors
AWOL risks, breaking out soars.
Seconds, minutes, hours pass

Morning music, silent lunch.

Smoke break's special to a whole bunch.

Are we mental? Doc, tell me.

What am I supposed to be?

18 Just a patient waiting through time

My mind's gone mad, I did no crime.

Questions, medicine, how do you feel?

How can this happen? Is this for real?

Waiting for your discharge date

With nothing to do, it's quite a wait.

Doc says you're well, and you can leave

Back to yourself. we hope. we believe.

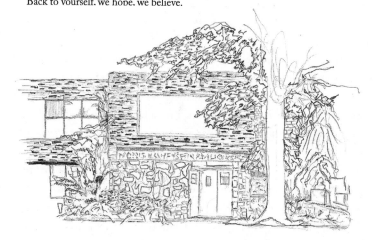

THE HOSPITAL

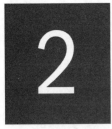

2

SO MANY QUESTIONS

Some people who have schizophrenia experience symptoms for a long time, possibly many years, before they get help. Other people seem to develop symptoms very suddenly. But as they begin to feel better, everyone has many questions. For this reason, this chapter discusses issues that often worry people as they begin to recover. Here are the most frequently asked questions, with answers by our team at Zucker Hillside Hospital. If you have more questions, write them down and discuss them with the people treating you. You will also find more information in the chapters that follow.

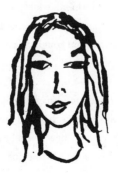

SASHA

Special contributors: Julia Becker, M.D. and Delbert Robinson, M.D.

SASHA: I came from a dysfunctional family. All my life I was transferred from one foster home to another and in and out of institutions. I didn't know my mother when I was young. I lived in an institution run by nuns until I was seven.

Now I am a 35-year-old woman with a 7-year-old son. I was a corrections officer making $40,000 a year. I was having suicidal thoughts because my life got me upset. I overdosed, so my stomach was pumped and I was referred for counseling.

I lost my job due to my psychosis and was placed in a psychiatric hospital where I was treated for schizophrenia. I had hallucinations: seeing people that looked like animals and horses with human heads; voices saying, "Sasha, how could you leave your son?" Other times they would say, "Leave him. He'd be better off without you." I was a compulsive cleaner, washing everything with Lysol every day. There was something strange about my face, but I don't remember. I used to masturbate a lot during that time. I thought somebody was talking through my mouth. I would polish my nails every day a different color. If I heard a voice when I was sitting on the bus, I would try to read a book. It sounded like the voice was next to me.

QUESTION:

What's happening to me?

ANSWER:

When you came into the hospital you were experiencing symptoms caused by a chemical imbalance in the brain. These are symptoms of a psychotic illness, just as a fever and coughing are symptoms of the flu. See the Symptom List in chapter 4.

GENEVIVE: They never told me I was sick until I left the hospital. If I'd been told that it was an illness, and they had explained the nature of the illness, that would have helped. I knew I was hearing the voices, but how come I was hearing them? And why did I think that even my mother was going to poison me?

QUESTION:

Am I the only one?

ANSWER:

Schizophrenia is a brain disorder that affects one percent of the population of the world. That means that there are over two million people in the United States alone who have schizophrenia. That's a lot of people. You are definitely not alone.

21

SHARON: I always felt like I was different from everybody else, always had to be in special education, always needed special attention. I wanted to be normal like everyone else. I hated the fact that when I was younger I had to take medicine because I was a hyperactive kid. All of a sudden they tell me I have an illness called schizophrenia. It made me feel ashamed of myself, like I couldn't do anything right like a normal person.

QUESTION:

Why me?

ANSWER:

Why this illness happens to one person and not another is still unknown. A number of researchers are investigating different possible causes of schizophrenia, but for now the exact cause is unknown. We know that schizophrenia's onset is usually between adolescence and age thirty-nine, but sometimes it affects younger or older people. We know that schizophrenia is not contagious. Although schizophrenia and other kinds of mental illness can run in families, we do not believe it is caused by family interaction. It is possible that there is a combination of causes at work. But no matter how this disease develops, it is important to remember that schizophrenia is an illness, and no one is responsible for causing it.

MARCUS: "Why is this happening to me and not to anyone else?" You were doing so good in the beginning and you didn't have any problems at all and all of a sudden this hits you and you wonder, "Why did this happen to me?" I thought about it a lot, but after a while you get over it. The medication and the groups help.

QUESTION:

Why now?

ANSWER:

Most people who develop schizophrenia do so in their late teens to mid-twenties. Many people have wondered about why things seem to be going along just fine and then suddenly there it is: schizophrenia. What we do know is that the brain continues to grow until the late teenage years. At that time it begins to go through a pruning process, like cutting back the branches of a tree when it gets too large and unruly. One thought is that something goes wrong in the pruning. But that is only one idea. Scientists are learning much more about the developing brain than ever before and hope to answer this question in the future.

QUESTION:

Can schizophrenia be cured?

ANSWER:

Schizophrenia is an illness that can be treated, but there is no cure at this time. In this way it is like diabetes or high blood pressure: it requires careful monitoring and treatment. Recovery is a slow process that usually takes many months. As with any other illness, each person's recovery is different. But most people experiencing schizophrenia for the first time respond well to medication. In time, many return to school or work, make friends, date, marry, and enjoy life again.

BEN: The first four times I was hospitalized, to me that was the learning process. For me it had to be, because if it wasn't then this illness would be lifelong. I learned what my illness was and to live with it, what I had to do. It took four hospitalizations, but the main thing is to take my medication.

RESEARCH FINDINGS

Will I Get Better?

People with first-episode schizophrenia or schizoaffective disorder have very high rates of response to medication treatment. Nine out of ten people with first-episode schizophrenia or schizoaffective disorder get *substantially* better with treatment; the others usually have *some* improvement despite continued symptoms. —Delbert Robinson, M.D.

QUESTION:

How is schizophrenia treated?

ANSWER:

Most people are treated for the first time in the hospital. While you are in the hospital you are in a safe place. The first task of the psychiatrists is to interview you in order to get a good picture of your symptoms. Asking you questions is the only way to find out what is wrong. Learning about your symptoms is like taking your temperature when you have the flu. Then your doctor may order lab tests or other tests such as a CAT scan or MRI to eliminate other possible disorders that might be causing the symptoms. Next your doctor usually prescribes medication. You are watched for any side effects, and the medication is adjusted depending upon how well you respond to it. It usually takes a while for symptoms to be adequately controlled. Once you are feeling better and the psychiatrist believes you are ready, you will be discharged. How long this takes varies for each person.

After discharge you will begin treatment with a psychiatrist and therapist or you may join a day program, which will provide intensive treatment to you as an outpatient. You will attend groups for therapy and receive help to get you ready to resume your life. You will also have access to a psychiatrist and a nurse to deal with any problems you might have with your medication. You may also have an individual therapist and a case manager. A case manager is someone who helps you with problems you might encounter after being discharged from the hospital, such as finding a place to live or getting benefits. When you leave the day program you will continue to see a psychiatrist and therapist, but less frequently. Since there is currently no cure for schizophrenia, you will need to continue to see your doctor regularly. Your need to see the psychiatrist and therapist will probably decrease as you improve.

VANESSA: I know my sister went through the same thing. She has schizophrenia and she was telling me that it doesn't happen to everybody. Some people don't expect it to happen to them. But it happened to her. She had similar reactions to what I had. She told me not to be afraid, that the medication would help me, and as long as I continued therapy that would help also.

QUESTION:
What about medication?
ANSWER:
The medicines that help eliminate psychotic symptoms are called antipsychotic medications. These work to decrease the chemical imbalance that is

causing symptoms. They are not addictive.

The psychiatrist gradually adjusts the medication so that you are getting the best dose for your individual needs. Since each person's body metabolizes medicine differently, it often takes several months to find the right dose for you. For a more complete explanation of how antipsychotic medications work, see chapter 8.

JEFF: Sometimes I think, "Why am I taking the medication, because I am not having a hard time?" But they say if you stop taking it you will have a relapse. I don't want to have any problems. It's kind of nice not having problems. They say I am taking it so I don't get into any psychotic moods.

RESEARCH FINDINGS

How Long Does It Take?

Most people have some improvement within one or two weeks of starting medication treatment. People continue to improve for a long time after that. The average length of medication treatment before the delusions and hallucinations totally go away is around two months. *Don't get discouraged too soon. Give the treatment time to work.* —Delbert Robinson, M.D.

The thermostat in your house keeps the temperature from getting too hot or too cold. The medicine works in a similar way. It regulates the chemicals of the brain so that they stay in the "comfortable zone."

QUESTION:

What are the side effects of medication, and should I be worried about them?

ANSWER:

Side effects are unwanted results of taking medication. Some people experience severe side effects, while others have mild side effects or none at all. Some common side effects of antipsychotic medications are weight gain, restlessness, tiredness, drooling, and muscle stiffness.

Some side effects decrease as your body adjusts to the medication. For instance, drooling and tiredness usually improve with time. However, it is important to *complain* to your doctor about any problems so adjustments or changes can be made. For example, don't be embarrassed to tell your doctor if you experience lowered sex drive. Medication adjustments can help, but *only* your doctor can safely make adjustments or changes to your medication. For additional information on side effects, see chapters 8 and 10.

RESEARCH FINDINGS

Do the Medications Have Side Effects?

Each of the medications has potential side effects. You should discuss with your doctor the potential side effects of the specific medication you are taking. If you experience anything that you think may be a side effect, be sure to bring this up with your doctor. Many medication side effects can be lessened or eliminated, but your doctor needs to know about them in order to help you. People with untreated side effects are more likely to stop their medications and thereby have a relapse. —Delbert Robinson, M.D.

NEW SIDE EFFECT FINDINGS

Increased Cholesterol and Insulin Levels

Most people beginning treatment today take one of the newer medications that have been developed to have fewer side effect problems. Unfortunately, some of these newer medications, such as olanzapine, clozapine, risperidone, quetiapine, ziprasidone, and aripiprazole, may cause metabolic problems.

There are two metabolic problems of concern: high cholesterol and increased insulin levels. For most people the metabolic problems are the result of weight gain that stresses the body in ways that cause the increased cholesterol and insulin levels. *This means it is important to have your cholesterol and insulin levels checked by your medical doctor every six months. And it means being extra careful to exercise and eat low-fat and low-calorie foods.* See chapter 11 for diet and exercise recommendations.

AMBER: The first medication they put me on was clozapine. I had a lot of side effects. I drooled a lot, and at times I was constipated. I had to have weekly blood tests to test the white blood cell count, and I didn't like the black-and-blue marks the needles gave me. I told my doctor about that, and she decided to switch me to another medicine called olanzapine. It has been working out great. I don't drool as much, and I don't have the constipation. It still makes me drowsy when I take it at night. But it helps me go to sleep, and it's been working out for me. I haven't had any symptoms since I was on Low III two years ago.

QUESTION:

How will the medication affect pregnancy?

ANSWER:

For females: If you decide to become pregnant, you should discuss it with your psychiatrist, who will advise you of your options. By planning carefully, you will be able to decrease risks to your unborn child.

For males: At this time there are no known risks to a child whose father is taking an antipsychotic medication at the time of conception. However, males on medication may have difficulty with sexual performance.

SAM: I had zero, less than zero, sexual interest when I was twenty-four on Prolixin. I didn't tell the doctor for two years.

QUESTION:

Can I ever go off my medication?

ANSWER:

Eliminating the psychotic symptoms requires taking antipsychotic medication. Even when the symptoms are gone, the medication continues to work to prevent the chemical imbalance in your brain from returning. For example, people with diabetes take medicine and adjust their diets in order to keep their blood sugar controlled. This prevents flare-ups and complications in the long run. Likewise, if you have schizophrenia, it is important to take the medications and work with the doctors not only to treat the symptoms but also to stay well.

Other factors involved in staying well include sleeping regularly, eating well, and getting exercise. Keeping stress levels low is also essential. Relapse is not good for you, and it feels awful. It is very disruptive to your life; you may lose your place in school or at work. It upsets people who care about you and adds to your hospital bills. Most important, sometimes people do not recover as well after several relapses.

BUCK: I thought I could live my life without taking medication, but I ended up in the hospital again. Then it got worse. I started losing my concentration and my memory got bad. That's when I finally realized I had to take the medication.

27

JEFF: The doctors say that 98 percent of the people who stop taking their medication go back into the hospital. So I take it. I don't want to have problems like that. Such a large number of people relapsed; I don't want to be a part of that. I want to be doing okay, just taking the meds.

QUESTION:

What if I refuse to take medication?

ANSWER:

If the medical team believes you are a danger to yourself or to other people, they will bring your case to a judge. The judge will decide whether you must remain in the hospital and take medication. If you are not in the hospital and you appear to be in danger of hurting yourself or others, anyone can contact the police to begin the treatment process. It is always in your own best interests to be a voluntary patient and work with your treatment team.

RESEARCH FINDINGS

Once I Get Better, Will My Symptoms Ever Return?

The medications improve symptoms but don't cure the disease. Maintenance medication decreases the risk of relapse. People who take maintenance medication have one fifth the risk of relapse of people who do not take maintenance medication. —Delbert Robinson, M.D.

QUESTION:

How do they know it is schizophrenia?

ANSWER:

Often, once the doctor gets a history of symptoms, he or she can give a clear diagnosis. Sometimes, at the beginning, it is harder to tell exactly what is wrong. For instance, schizoaffective disorder is one form of schizophrenia, but it can look a lot like bipolar disorder (also known as manic depression). The doctor may need more time to make a diagnosis in such cases. For additional information on diagnosing schizophrenia, see chapter 6.

ZELDA: Doctors and therapists made their decision based upon observations of my situation—paranoia, mixed-up thinking, delusions, depression. These symptoms were real. So, if these signs all point to schizophrenia, I suppose I've got a case. Generally, that's one description of who I am today—but that's not the only one. I don't fit that neatly into a box.

3 HOW THE BRAIN WORKS

When the brain is healthy, it enables us to think, to learn, to feel, to work, and to move. But the brain is a complex piece of equipment, and sometimes it doesn't function properly. Imagine a computer that has a serious problem with its hard drive. When this happens, the computer will act in unpredictable ways. The same is true for the brain—if the equipment breaks down or malfunctions, our thoughts, feelings, and behavior can become distorted. It might feel as if someone else is in control or as if your brain has a mind of its own.

Feeling like you have lost control is frightening. But remember, you as a person have not changed. You will be the same person when the equipment problem is corrected.

SAMANTHA: I'm forty-five years old now. Five years ago I was diagnosed with schizophrenia. Prior to that time I led a relatively normal life as a mother, wife, and breadwinner with a house in Seattle. Two years before my diagnosis, symptoms of schizophrenia started appearing and continued to grow: poor concentration, extreme distraction, irrational decisions, delusions, and auditory hallucinations. At the time I joined a church group. Following my association with this group I snapped, and everything got worse.

My life completely decomposed. I couldn't concentrate on a simple job. I resigned from an excellent job that I had. I tried to go back to school

Special contributor: Handan Gunduz-Bruce, M.D.

with the idea that I was going to become a professional dancer, which was a major delusion. I also had a delusion of thinking I was a missionary in Seattle and led my life with both of these grand delusions. I spent a semester dancing, wearing nothing but tights and leotards. I took five dance classes a day. Now remember, I was thirty-seven years old then. People don't leave great jobs to go into dance at age thirty-seven. I thought I was going to be the star dancer on the stage. My professors realized something was amiss, and after a semester at college I was asked to leave.

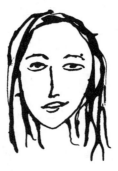

SAMANTHA

I tried to go back to work again, unsuccessfully. I started having very bad problems with distractibility, wandering around, doing my own type of thing on the job, and was fired. Then I went into the next phase of my delusions, which was thinking I was a visionary.

My husband divorced me. I agreed to move out of my house. The attorney assisting me in our divorce settlement did not help. This resulted in no financial resources. So I lived in a one-bedroom apartment in an isolated part of town, walking thirteen and fourteen miles a day. I was roaming, walking, hiking, and doing good deeds whenever I came across them. On my walks I imagined voices in my head—people I knew from the church group—telling me to do these deeds. For example, I was on one of my walks on a hot, sunny day when I came across some kids playing ball without supervision. One kid fell down and hurt his knee. I thought it was my responsibility to bring him home and get medical assistance. And that's what I did. Of course it was absolutely none of my business what these children were doing. When I returned the child to his mother I was verbally attacked. The police were called to come and arrest me for kidnapping.

I ate rice with chopped-up brussels sprouts for breakfast and dinner. I slept once every three days, did not see my daughter all month, and wore black hiking shoes, which caused my feet to bleed. I baked chocolate chip cookies every day, and that is what I lived on.

31

My unemployment and assistance from Seattle were not renewed. I had an eye infection that was untreated because I had no medical insurance. I had no resources to fall back on, none whatsoever. I had been seeing a counselor who was of no help. My cousin realized something was wrong and helped me make a decision to call for an ambulette to take me to a county hospital. I was in that hospital for two weeks. I didn't cooperate with the doctors, the staff, or the program and begged my parents to help bail me out. My parents brought me back to New York. Then they began to realize that something was wrong.

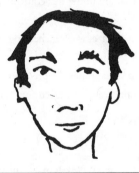

MARK

MARK: It was probably the best time of my life. I was doing very well in school, very well. I was looking good, had a lot of energy, and was very happy. Unfortunately, things got away from me. I can't say I had a reason, but they just did. The line between reality and dream gradually faded.

The biggest thing I remember is that I had no warning. It just happened: time and space distortion, things moving slower or faster, hallucinations—things looking bigger, stretching out, faces warping. I could not think logically. I was caught up in emotion. The best way I can explain is to say it's like when you are dreaming; things don't make sense, but you accept them. But when you dream, the brain cuts off from your body. I was awake, but I would act based on the "dream." I would cry because

I felt like crying. It was like every drug you could do, but I wasn't doing drugs and I wasn't in a dream. I was awake, but I thought it was all real. Then I kind of repented. I started looking for explanations. Unfortunately, the first thing that should have—but didn't—come into my head was that I should see a doctor.

WHAT THE BRAIN DOES

Samantha and Mark's brains were not functioning the way they had been before their symptoms appeared. Understanding how the brain works helps us understand why this might happen.

Basically, the brain is in charge of:

- automatic functions required for survival, such as heartbeat and breathing
- motor functions that are under our control, such as throwing a ball and writing
- sensory processes, such as seeing, hearing, smelling, tasting, and perceiving pain or touch
- feeling states, such as happiness, depression, anxiety, and fear
- intellectual functions, such as attention, concentration, learning, and memory.

PARTS OF THE BRAIN

The two major parts of our nervous system are the central nervous system and the peripheral nervous system. The central nervous system is made up of the cerebral hemispheres (cerebrum) and the spinal cord. The peripheral nervous system is made up of nerve cells extending from the spinal cord.

Figure 3.3 shows the gross anatomy of the cerebral hemispheres (excluding the cerebellum and spinal cord). The cerebrum consists of five parts: the frontal lobe, the parietal lobe, the temporal lobe, the occipital lobe, and the limbic lobe.

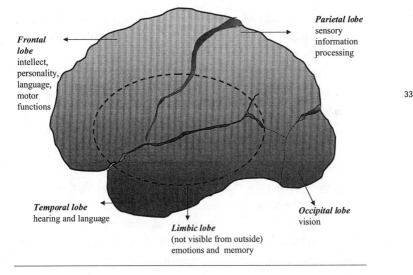

Frontal lobe
intellect,
personality,
language,
motor
functions

Parietal lobe
sensory
information
processing

Temporal lobe
hearing and language

Limbic lobe
(not visible from outside)
emotions and memory

Occipital lobe
vision

FIGURE 3.3

CEREBRAL HEMISPHERES

The *frontal lobe* is primarily responsible for the intellectual functions, personality, and some language and motor functions.

The *parietal lobe* processes sensory information.

The *temporal lobe* functions in hearing and language.

The *occipital lobe* plays a role in vision.

The *limbic lobe* has a role in memory and emotional processing.

HOW THE BRAIN SENDS MESSAGES

Neurons

The brain contains about 10 billion nerve cells known as neurons. Each of these neurons communicates with more than a thousand other neurons at connections between them called synapses. There are three parts of a neuron: the *soma (cell body)*, the *axon*, and the *dendrite*.

The *cell body* is star shaped, with many protrusions on its surface called dendrites. One dendrite, called the axon, is particularly long, like a cable. The cell body contains the nucleus and the other essential components that are necessary for the metabolism of the cell. It receives electrical signals from the many dendrites on its surface and, like a computer, processes all these incoming signals to produce an outgoing signal that travels down its axon.

Like an electrical cable, the *axon* carries an electrical signal along its length. It can be quite long, as much as several hundred times the length of the cell body. For example, a motor neuron that carries information from the brain down to a leg muscle can be 40 inches long.

34

The *dendrite* receives signals and sends them to the cell body. Two neurons communicate at the point where an axon from one neuron comes very close to the dendrite of another. This region is called a *synapse*. The space between the tip of the axon—the *synaptic terminal*—and the dendrite is called the synaptic cleft.

The electrical impulse that arrives at the synaptic terminal of the first neuron leads to a release of a chemical substance called a *neurotransmitter* into the synaptic cleft. When the neurotransmitter reaches the dendrites of the second neuron and attaches to receptors on them, this triggers the second neuron to send an electrical impulse.

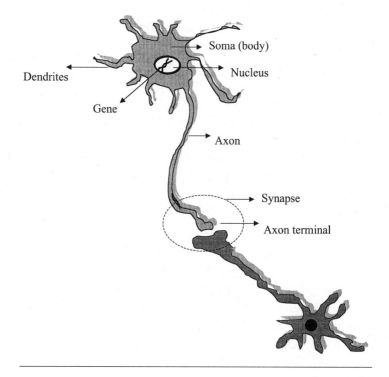

FIGURE 3.4

STRUCTURE OF A NEURON

Neurotransmitters

In order for the different parts of the brain to communicate, the neurons that connect them must be able to send their electrical signals properly. This depends on the ability of the neurotransmitters at each synapse to relay signals from one neuron to the next. Some brain disorders are due to a defect in the ability of one neuron's neurotransmitter to stimulate another neuron to act.

There are different kinds of neurotransmitters. Some are found throughout the brain; others are found only in certain parts. Several neurotransmitters are thought to play a role in causing the symptoms of schizophrenia. One of them is called dopamine, and another glutamate.

Dopamine is mostly found in the basal ganglia, a region of the brain located in the base of the cerebrum. Most of the older medications used to treat psychotic symptoms work by reducing the activity of the dopamine in this area of the brain.

Glutamate is present all over the brain, and it is a major neurotransmitter that causes excitation on a neuronal level. Several recent genetic studies suggest that genes that play a role in glutamate regulation may be abnormal in schizophrenia.

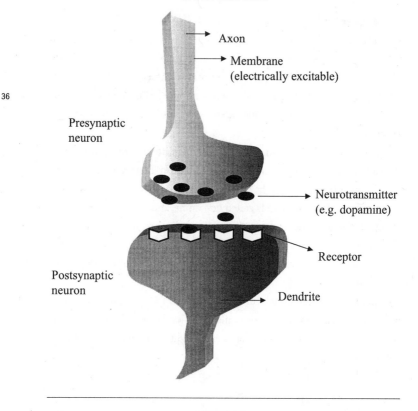

FIGURE 3.5

STRUCTURE OF A SYNAPSE

There are special proteins on the surface of the receiving neuron called receptors. They receive the neurotransmitters coming from the sending neuron. When a neurotransmitter attaches to a receptor, the receptor responds by setting a chain of events into motion. For example, a receptor may start a process whereby the neuron will release its own neurotransmitter or secrete a hormone, depending on the neuron's specific function.

The complexity of the brain is due to the very large number of connections among the brain lobes as well as within each of them. These connections carry information between different parts of the brain as it performs its operations. Therefore, when one part of the brain is affected by a disease, several other parts can be affected as well. For example, a person who suffers a stroke may have muscle weakness, difficulty with speech, and feelings of depression. A person with schizophrenia may have poor concentration and memory problems; they may also experience unusual sensations such as hearing voices, seeing visions, or having unusual thought patterns.

> The brain is like the Internet. Signals get sent and are received among many parts of a complicated system.

Let's look at a very simplified example of the brain at work. Your friend accidentally steps on your foot. The nerve cell (neuron) in your foot sends the feeling of pain on to the nerve cell in your brain. But there is a space (synapse) between the two cells. To move the message, the neuron needs a messenger. The messenger, dopamine—a kind of neurotransmitter—carries the impulse from the axon across the synapse to the dendrite of the next neuron. There a receptor is waiting to attach itself to the dopamine. It carries the message to the home base (cell body). The message gets interpreted, and you feel pain in your foot.

Now, what if there is a chemical imbalance? What if there are too few or too many dopamine or receptor chemicals? Imagine a toy train set. Too little power and the train stops. Too much power and the train flies off the track. That is what happens when you are experiencing symptoms of psychosis. The message gets confused. You might think your friend purposely stepped on you.

Additional information about the brain:

The Scientific American Day in the Life of Your Brain, by Judith Horstman (Jossey-Bass, 2009).

Brain Basics: Know Your Brain, National Institute of Neurological Disorders and Stroke. Available free at www.ninds.nih.gov/disorders/brain_basics/know_your_brain.htm or call 1-800-352-9424.

The Life and Death of a Neuron, Brain Basics, National Institute of Neurological Disorders and Stroke. Available free at www.ninds.nih.gov/disorders/brain_basics/ninds_neuron.htm or call 1-800-352-9424.

4

WHAT IS SCHIZOPHRENIA?

Schizophrenia is a disease of the brain that affects about one percent of the population. It affects males and females equally, often occurring between adolescence and young adulthood. It disturbs how the brain functions to differing degrees and in different ways. These disturbances, called symptoms, can include delusions, confused thinking, and hallucinations.

We know that schizophrenia is a medical illness. We also know that it is not contagious. A number of researchers are investigating different possible causes of schizophrenia, but for now the exact cause is unknown. There may be a combination of factors at work (see chapter 5). But no matter how this disease develops, it is important to remember that schizophrenia is an illness of the brain and it is no one's fault. The brain is an organ like any other organ in the body, and it can get sick just like the heart, lungs, skin, kidneys, or other organs.

JACKIE: I was twenty-three. I went through a stressful situation, broke up with my boyfriend, and I was alone living in Colorado. I didn't have much family there, and I got very lonely. I started having anxiety attacks and panic attacks. I got very paranoid. I thought the whole world was out to get me. I stayed cooped up in my apartment, very rarely going outside. I didn't feel right. I just wanted to go home.

So eventually I decided to move back to New York. When I got home I moved in with my mother and started looking for waitressing jobs. Ev-

Special contributor: Julia Becker, M.D.

ery time I went to fill out an application I got paranoid. You had to fill out the part about previous convictions. I wasn't convicted, but I had been arrested for DWI in Colorado. So I never handed in the applications. I was searching for a job for months, but I was just too paranoid.

One time when I went into the city to look for a job I was taking the train, and there were these fires on the tracks. I thought I was on the train to hell. Eventually I became afraid to leave the house and stayed in the house every day, all day. My brother realized that what my mother had been telling him was true: something was very wrong. My brother asked me to come up to Connecticut and visit him. I took the train to go to the Port Authority, but the voices told me to get off and get on a different train. I found myself in Roslyn, feeling lost, and called my father to pick me up. So the next day I was determined to make it to Hartford, and I did get on the bus. I thought the man sitting next to me urinated. There were a lot of strange smells on that bus. I started getting this ringing in my ears. It was so loud.

And then I started hearing voices. I mainly heard the voice of my ex-boyfriend. I thought he was some kind of god or some kind of devil. I wasn't sure which. I thought he was doing telepathy with me from Denver to New York. So I started listening to the voices. When it came to getting dressed, the voices told me when to put something on and when not to. I was listening to every word they said.

Eventually voices of other people I knew from the past came into my head. I was not eating at all, but whenever I tried to eat the food would come back up. When I slept it seemed as if I were still hearing the voices in my dreams. A lot of times they woke me up. Up until I got treatment, I thought there were a hundred people watching me 24/7. So I had to shower very quickly because it felt like a lot of people were watching me. I did shower, but it was because I was afraid, paranoid about being clean. I wasn't eating and I wasn't talking to anybody. One time a friend tried to take me out with our friends, but I just sat there the whole night.

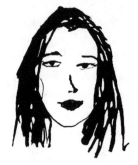

JACKIE

There was one time that was really scary. I was hallucinating that I was in this big room with a thousand people and all those people were watching me shower. A lot of times I was thinking that because I was hearing my ex-boyfriend's voice saying I was killing him. So I started to have thoughts of suicide. Somehow I was hurting all these people, so I had to die to save them. I wasn't really suicidal, but I was thinking what I should do to end my life. I thought my mother was evil. She looked different to me. I thought she was trying to replace me with a girl that I had problems with in high school. I thought she was taking her on as a daughter and giving me up. I had hallucinations that this girl was manipulating me and trying to switch places with me. In the hallucination it felt as if she were doing some kind of magic to switch places with me.

My mother tried to get me to go to the hospital, but I refused. So my brother made a deal with me. He would take the bus with me up to Hartford and back to see if it would clear up the voices in my head. I thought that was the solution. If he did that but the voices stayed, I would agree to go to the hospital. So we took the bus up and back and nothing changed; the voices were still there. They took me to the hospital the next day.

SYMPTOMS OF SCHIZOPHRENIA

Schizophrenia is a disease that involves a group of symptoms that usually occur in young people for no apparent reason. Doctors do not yet know precisely what causes this illness. It is not curable, but it can be treated with medication.

Schizophrenia affects thinking, feeling, movement, and behavior. These are all regulated by the brain, an organ that orchestrates many thousands of activities at once. For instance, think about all of the things the brain must coordinate in order for you to ride a bicycle. Your legs have to pedal to make the bike move forward. Your hands have to hold the handlebars to steer. Meanwhile, your eyes are watching the street for obstacles. Your heart beats faster when you pedal up a steep hill. These are just a few of the tasks your brain oversees.

When the brain is assaulted by an illness such as schizophrenia, its usual processing can be disturbed in several ways. We divide these symptoms into three categories: positive symptoms, negative symptoms, and cognitive symptoms.

Positive Symptoms

Positive symptoms are the presence of sensations, beliefs, and behaviors that would not normally occur. These are the symptoms that are very noticeable and of which people are most aware.

DISTURBANCES OF THOUGHT PROCESSES Your thought processes can be disrupted so that one thought does not directly relate to the previous thought. Or the mind can play tricks, making things seem real even though they are not.

It can feel like certain alien thoughts have been physically put into your mind (thought insertion) or as if something or someone has pulled one of your thoughts out of your mind (thought withdrawal). Your thoughts may be interrupted in midstream, as if something is preventing your ability to think clearly. This can make it very difficult to have a conversation. It might also seem like your thoughts are being broadcast out loud so that other people can hear them.

DELUSIONS Delusions are beliefs that are not true. There are several different kinds of delusions. If you believe that people are trying to harm you even though this is not the case, you are suffering from a paranoid delusion. This can be a terrifying experience because it seems so real. Delusions of reference occur when things in the environment seem to be directly related to you even though they are not. For example, it may seem as if people are talking about you or special personal messages are being communicated to you through the TV, radio, or other media. Somatic delusions are erroneous beliefs about your body, for example, that a terrible physical illness exists or that something foreign is inside or passing through your body. Delusions of grandeur occur when you believe you are very special or have special powers and abilities. An example of a grandiose delusion is thinking you are a famous rock star.

HALLUCINATIONS When you hear, see, smell, taste, or feel something that is not really there, you are having a hallucination. There are five different kinds of hallucinations, one for each of our senses:

- auditory—hearing things that other people do not hear
- visual—seeing things that other people do not see
- olfactory—smelling things that other people do not smell
- tactile—feeling something touching your skin that is not there
- gustatory—tasting something that is not there.

FEELINGS Feelings are sometimes seriously affected by schizophrenia. Your emotions may be very erratic: on some occasions your mood may be better than usual and you may even feel extremely happy or silly; on other occasions you may feel extremely sad or depressed. You may feel that you are not real or alive. You may experience the sensation of having no feelings at all. Unfortunately, sometimes people with schizophrenia feel that they do not want to go on living.

It is extremely important to let your doctor and treatment team know how you are feeling. Though your situation may seem bad at one moment, it is temporary, and your symptoms are treatable. So share your concerns with your doctor.

MOVEMENTS There can be changes in the way you move: your movements can become very slow or very fast. On rare occasions, some people slow down so much that they do not move for long periods of time and someone has to help them feed themselves or get in and out of bed. This is called catatonia. Odd movements and unusual gestures or postures may be seen during the active phase of the illness. Imagined voices (auditory hallucinations) may be commanding a person to move a particular way. Sometimes people move in unusual ways because of delusional beliefs. For example, someone taps his feet to make people stop talking about him.

BEHAVIOR People suffering from schizophrenia may act in ways that are unusual for them. For instance, some people develop very poor judgment or behave in sexually inappropriate ways. Others may become threatening to those around them because of fears that they themselves may be harmed.

Negative Symptoms

Negative symptoms are the lack of important abilities. Some of these include:

- the inability to enjoy activities as much as before
- low energy
- a blank, blunted facial expression or having less lively facial movement or physical movement
- low motivation
- difficulty initiating activities
- inability to make friends or keep friends, or not caring to have friends.

Although at first glance these symptoms may seem less disruptive than the voices, strange thoughts, or delusions, they can affect your life significantly. Luckily, newer antipsychotic medications have been helpful in treating negative symptoms.

Cognitive Symptoms

Cognitive symptoms refer to difficulties with concentration and memory. They include:

- disorganized thinking
- slow thinking
- difficulty understanding
- poor concentration
- poor memory
- difficulty expressing thoughts
- difficulty integrating thoughts, feelings, and behavior.

When thinking, feeling, behavior, or movement is affected by this illness, it's hard not to feel confused and disturbed. Delusions and hallucinations can seem very real. It is no wonder that people who have schizophrenia believe so strongly in them. You may experience many of the symptoms mentioned, although probably not all of them. If you have any symptoms that are not listed here, talk to your doctor. He or she will be able to explain them individually.

SYMPTOM LIST

Hallucinations—sensory perceptions that have the compelling sense of reality of a true perception, but that occur without external stimulation of the relevant sensory organ
- auditory: hearing things that other people do not hear
- visual: seeing things that other people do not see
- olefactory: smelling things that other people do not smell
- tactile: feeling something touching your skin that is not there
- gustatory: tasting something that is not there

Delusions—false beliefs

Example: You think someone wants to hurt you even though this is not true.

Confused thinking—unclear or mixed-up thoughts

Unusual behavior—doing things that are strange

Example: You stand like a bird.

Change in feelings or unusual feelings—feeling about things very differently from how you used to feel

Difficulty doing everyday tasks—having a tough time with your usual routine

Example: You are unable to get out of bed or go to work.

Social isolation—spending most of the day alone or only with your family.

Additional information about schizophrenia and psychosis:

Me, Myself, and Them: A Firsthand Account of One Young Person's Experience with Schizophrenia, by Kurt Snyder, Raquel E. Gur, and Linda Wasmer Andrews (Oxford University Press, 2007)

Surviving Schizophrenia: A Manual for Families, Patients, and Providers, by E. Fuller Torrey (Harper, 2006)

The Quiet Room: A Journey Out of the Torment of Madness, by Lori Schiller and Amanda Bennett (Grand Central Publishing, 1996)

Understanding Mental Illness and Schizophrenia (DVD) (Information Television Network, 2006)

EPPIC Program in Australia: www.eppic.org.au

Early Psychosis Intervention Program in Canada: www.psychosissucks.ca/epi/

NARSAD Research: www.narsad.org/

MayoClinic.com: www.mayoclinic.com/

Texas Department of State Health Services: www.dshs.state.tx.us/mhprograms/
PtEd.shtm (English and Spanish)

NIMH: www.nimh.nih.gov/health/publications/schizophrenia/complete-index.
shtml (English and Spanish)

NAMI: www.nami.org/

WHY ME?

It is natural to want to know why this happened to you. Although there is no complete scientific explanation why some people develop schizophrenia, the same is true for many illnesses. There are many mysteries that scientists are just beginning to unravel.

Some people with schizophrenia wonder if they did something wrong that brought on this illness. Was there too much stress in their lives? Did they do too many street drugs? They often feel guilty or ashamed, angry or sad, even helpless. Remember not to blame yourself or your family. Stay up to date with the latest research findings.

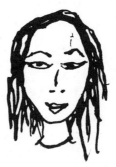

BETH

Special contributors: Handan Gunduz, M.D. and Anil Malhotra, M.D.

BETH: I was nineteen, and I was in college at the University of Buffalo. It was the beginning of my sophomore year. I remember bits and pieces of it. I remember my friends said that I was acting weird. I was dating somebody, and I thought we were going to get married. I was just not in reality at all. I was lying on my bed, and I was thinking there was a war going on. My roommates took me to the emergency room, and I stayed in the hospital for two weeks. Then they transferred me here. I never knew there was anything wrong with me. When they were doing testing I thought I was special, that people wanted to interview me, and that's why I was there. I was taking Haldol and Cogentin when I was upstate. Then I came to Hillside in a little bit better condition, still not understanding what was going on. I was there for a month or two and I couldn't finish up my semester at school. I don't think anybody had said the word *schizophrenia* when I was there. I was really upset afterward. I really didn't know what was happening. I thought I was on a cruise. I definitely had delusions of grandeur.

I wound up going to a local college and finished up my prerequisites for my program. I lost a whole year, and I was very upset about that. They just took me away from my school and my friends. I was furious. Then I had to apply to my program all over again, so I worked for another semester.

Nobody in my family has ever had a mental illness. I was a good kid. I always ask, "Why me?" I never thought it could happen to me. I still don't know. I just think it's not fair.

BIOLOGICAL CAUSES

Although the exact cause of schizophrenia is not known, it appears to be a biological disease. It is not caused by how someone is raised. We know that schizophrenia frequently runs in families. In other words, a person is more likely to develop schizophrenia if he or she has a relative with schizophrenia rather than no relatives with this illness. This indicates that genetic factors play a role.

Another factor that has been associated with developing schizophrenia is a history of obstetric complications. Many studies have shown that mothers of people with schizophrenia had more complications than average during their pregnancies, at birth, or right after birth. Decreased oxygen availability to the baby's brain around birth is known to damage certain regions of the brain that, later in life, play a role in its complex functions.

Some studies have indicated that viral and autoimmune mechanisms may be involved in risk factors for developing schizophrenia. After the 1957 flu epidemic, children born to mothers infected with flu in their second month of pregnancy were found to be twice as likely to develop schizophrenia as children whose mothers were not infected.

Some scientists are also expressing concern about marijuana use and schizophrenia. They believe that the chemicals in marijuana may change the way the brain develops, especially for younger teenagers. The effects of marijuana use on the brain continue to be explored in ongoing research.

These studies indicate that there may be problems in the way the brain matures that are due to genetics or to irregularities in the development of the brain. Although our knowledge about what causes schizophrenia is limited, with the advancement of scientific techniques, researchers are now able to design and conduct more powerful studies of this illness.

"Why Me?"

JACKIE: I went through a couple of years where I had a lot of regrets and I thought if I hadn't done certain things in my life it would never have happened to me. I blamed myself a lot. I also blamed my ex-boyfriend. I felt the way he treated me was the cause. Mainly I blamed myself for everything. It took me a couple of years to get over that.

THOMAS: Well, sometimes I think, "Why does this have to happen to me?" I am not really a bad person. I thought I was reasonably healthy. I used to think I did something bad, so I deserved it. Now I think there was no reason for this; it just happened.

AUDREY: At the start of the illness I would ask, "Why me?" Now I ask myself, "Why not me?"

BEAUX: "Why me?" is feeling sorry for yourself. It's uncontrollable.

BUCK: The first thing that I wanted to ask the doctor was why this happened to me. Sometimes I wonder if I did something wrong to deserve this illness. I don't know why it happened to me. I guess it's just part of life that you have to go through.

LUCINDA: Why not me? Worse could have happened. I could have been diagnosed with cancer. Schizophrenia is a treatable illness.

TABLE 5.1

Genetic Chance for Developing Schizophrenia

RELATIVE WITH SCHIZOPHRENIA	APPROXIMATE CHANCE OF DEVELOPING SCHIZOPHRENIA	APPROXIMATE CHANCE OF REMAINING FREE OF SCHIZOPHRENIA
Sibling	8%	92%
Twin (identical)	50%	50%
Twin (fraternal)	12%	88%
One Parent	12%	88%
Two Parents	40%	60%

ILAN: I think the "why me" for me came the second time around. The first time, being a religious person, I thought that I was being punished in some way or it was something that was supposed to happen. I thought it was good for me. "Even though I don't see it now," I told myself, "I'll understand it in the future." So in between the first day hospital and the second hospitalization I tried very hard to be more observant, very religious. So I was thinking, "Why me? What did I do this time that I deserve to come back?"

GARY: I remember asking myself "Why me?" after my discharge. It seemed like I said that for a good year.

MIKE: I never would have expected anything to happen to my mind. It was very unexpected and it was hard to deal with. I always questioned why I had to go through this. Was there a purpose behind it? Did I do anything to cause this to happen?

Now I know that I had nothing to do with getting this illness. I don't blame myself. I don't blame anyone else for this illness. It just happens.

WHY SOME PEOPLE DEVELOP SCHIZOPHRENIA

Schizophrenia is a biological illness. Scientists are not sure what causes it.

They believe it is related to genes, viruses, and problems at birth. They also are looking closely at differences in brain structure and environmental factors, such as early marijuana use and life stressors. Scientists do not believe schizophrenia is a result of how your parents raise you or a weakness in your character.

Psychiatric Genetic Research

Psychiatry is one of the youngest fields of medicine. As a result, our understanding of psychiatric disorders is still in its infancy. There are numerous mysteries about the underlying biological processes involved. There are also questions about treatment. One of the most puzzling questions commonly asked by patients is "Where did this come from?" or "How did I get this?" Nature versus nurture is one of the oldest scientific debates that attempts to answer this question. Essentially, the controversy is about whether we are influenced more by the biological traits we inherit from our parents or by the environment in which we are raised. One of the reasons this is such a difficult question to answer is that people in research studies usually share both similar biological traits and similar backgrounds. This makes it hard to separate the influence of biology from the influence of the environment.

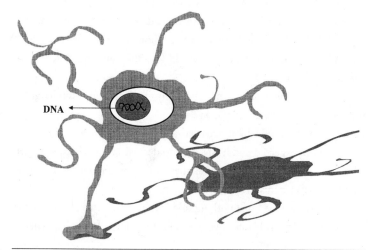

DNA

FIGURE 5.2

NEURON AND DNA

When we look at the influence of biology we are talking about genes, which are the basic unit of heredity. Genes are inherited in pairs, 23 pairs in all. The field of genetics attempts to understand how a person's characteristics and traits may be inherited biologically from his or her parents. Characteristics can be physical (for example, eye color, hair color, height) or behavioral (for example, musical ability). Genetic studies of psychiatric illness attempt to track how frequently psychiatric illnesses occur within families. They also attempt to identify which genes might be responsible for transmitting an illness from one generation to another. Studies of monozygotic twins, otherwise known as identical twins, were among the first genetic studies. Identical twins were studied because they are 100 percent genetically similar, while other pairs of family members are only 50 percent genetically similar. In order to focus on the influence of the environment, researchers turned to twin adoption studies. These studies looked at identical twins who had been adopted away from their biological parents and raised separately. However, because adoptive families are often carefully chosen so that the twins will grow up in similar environments, this makes it difficult to distinguish between environmental and hereditary influences. Therefore, these studies were not able to offer a lot of additional insight. Another type of study is the high-risk study, in which children with at least one ill parent, usually the mother, are studied over many years to identify risk factors and early signs of an illness. This type of research is important in helping us to identify potential causes of an illness.

Although an illness "runs in a family," that does not necessarily mean that the cause of that illness is purely genetic. Environmental influences such as stress, a virus, birth complications, and nutrition can help determine whether one will or will not develop a particular illness even if a genetic predisposition is present. One of the current theories is that the interaction of genetics and environment causes a psychiatric illness to emerge. According to this *interactionist theory*, individuals who develop a psychiatric illness are genetically predisposed to it, but environmental or developmental factors may trigger its onset. For example, among identical twins the probability that one twin will develop schizophrenia if the other twin has already been affected is about 46 percent (C. A. Prescott and I. I. Gottesman, "Genetically Mediated Vulnerability to Schizophrenia," Psychiatric Clinics of North America 16 [1993]: 245–267). This leads us to

51

wonder why the other 54 percent do not develop schizophrenia, whether the twins grow up together or apart. If genetics were the whole story, then we would expect both twins to be equally affected all the time. This implies that more than simple genetic inheritance contributes to the illness.

Newer types of genetic research examine the relationship between a person's genetic makeup and the characteristics they display. An important concept is that one's *genotype*, the specific genetic information inherited from one's parents, does not necessarily dictate one's *phenotype*, one's observable physical and behavioral characteristics. In other words, we are all coded with some genetic information that is never expressed in an observable way. This might occur for different reasons. Sometimes it may be because we have two different sets of genes, dominant and recessive, that give the body opposite sets of instructions about how to develop. Dominant genes hide the presence of recessive genes, and we never see the genetic information those genes contain, although it is still there. Another reason this might occur is that phenotype may not be linked to one gene alone but may reflect the influence of many genes. For example, linkage studies have been used to identify genes responsible for inherited human disease. These studies try to match particular traits to specific positions on the chromosomes that carry the genes. Association studies explore the relationship between specific traits (such as the presence or absence of an illness) and particular genes. These studies look at the DNA, the genetic material of which genes are made. DNA is collected from large groups of people with schizophrenia and their families and is then compared to the DNA of people without the trait. Researchers are now beginning to identify genes that might be implicated in the development of different psychiatric disorders, including schizophrenia. —Anil Malhotra, M.D., Unit of Molecular Psychiatry, Zucker Hillside Hospital

"My Background, My Genes"

SAM: I felt I was doing everything right. I know I was doing the job better than others. I didn't do anything wrong. I was moral and religious. I still am. I'll never be like the other kids in school. If I get married and have children, they may have it.

AMBER: I sometimes wonder why this incident happened to me. I was under a lot of stress. At the time I was looking for a job. It was a very stressful time for me, and that could be a reason why this happened. Also, my uncle had a mental disorder. I don't know exactly what it was, so I can't say if it was a genetic thing or not.

BUDDY: I used to think about "why me," but coming here made me understand that I'm not the one to blame. It is just something that I had no control over, that I was born with.

ALEXIS: I know that this is hereditary and I accept that.

SHARON: I know it's not my fault. I think the illness was caused by my background, my genes.

JAMES: I thought, "Why me?" when I came out of the hospital, and I still do to this day. I wondered, but then once I got out and I remembered what some of the doctors were telling me, that it was a chemical imbalance, that made it much better. I never thought it was my mother and father or my family that drove me to get sick, although I did have some stressful times in my life. I know we all do. I guess we all have different degrees that we can handle, but once the doctors told me it was a chemical imbalance I never believed it was caused by stress.

VANESSA: I couldn't understand why it happened to me. I was working. I had a nice job, two children. I just didn't understand why, what was going on.

ONE GENOME, 22,000 GENES, 23 PAIRS OF CHROMOSOMES

The human genome is how we describe all of a person's genetic makeup.

The genome has approximately 22,000 genes.

Genes are like codes that tell the body how it will look and act.

The 22,000 genes are contained within 23 pairs of chromosomes.

We inherit our chromosomes in pairs, 23 from each parent.

We inherit genes that carry traits that may make us vulnerable to a disease.

Sometimes there are changes in the gene structure during the process of copying genes from the parents' genes to the developing embryo.

There may be other reasons genes are altered that are now being explored.

Recent research is findng very small changes in genes may also play a role in developing schizophrenia.

Research continues to try to understand:

- which genes or combination of genes play a role in schizophrenia
- the interaction between genes and the environment
- who is at risk for developing schizophrenia

- what is going wrong for the genes involved.

For additional information about genetics and schizophrenia:
DukeHealth.org:

    www.dukehealth.org/health_library/news/schizophrenia_genetics_evidence_
fingers_emerging_class_of_culprits

Schizophrenia.com: http://www.schizophrenia.com/hypo.php

"The Genetics of Schizophrenia: Chromosomal Deletions, Attentional Disturbances, and Spectrum Boundaries," by Kenneth S. Kendler (*The American Journal of Psychiatry*, 2003): ajp.psychiatryonline.org/cgi/content/full/160/9/1549

6 DIAGNOSING SCHIZOPHRENIA

Some illnesses can be detected with an x-ray or a blood test, but diagnosing schizophrenia is more complicated. Doctors gather information about you from you and people close to you, then decide whether your symptoms fit with a diagnosis of schizophrenia or some other psychiatric disorder.

There are many psychiatric illnesses that share some of the same symptoms. For example, delusions or hallucinations often occur with severe depression as well as with schizophrenia. For this reason, making an accurate diagnosis can take a few days or even a few months.

To complicate the task further, there are also several different types of schizophrenia disorders. In time your doctors will be able to identify which type of schizophrenia you have. This will help them plan your treatment.

BUDDY: I was seventeen years old when I first had symptoms. My imagination started running wild in the summer two years ago. I was working, doing an internship at a community paper. I started getting a lot of ideas. I didn't have control of my thoughts. Everything was going too fast.

There were times I would get up in the middle of the night with an idea, constantly thinking, my thoughts running wild. It started to affect me at my job. I was working on the computer when I felt something going wrong in my head. I was speaking to the publisher, who said every-

Special contributors: Handan Gunduz, M.D. and Julia Becker, M.D.

thing was okay. I guess it was an anxiety attack. I kept going back and forth to the computer until I told myself I had to go home. That was the first episode I recall. A few days later at work I had another anxiety attack. I felt people were talking about me behind my back; they were out to get me because I wasn't doing a good job. I got into some arguments with some co-employees. I wasn't able to focus.

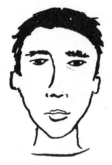

BUDDY

One day I had to go out in the yard and sweep, and my mind was just wandering. I would sweep one spot for a long time, not conscious of what I was doing. It was like I couldn't focus on the job. The pinnacle came a week before school started in my senior year. At my job they left me alone cooking hamburgers on the grill, and there was a rush. I was sweating scared because I didn't know what I was doing. I told the supervisor I needed a break, that I had family problems, a lot of things on my mind. He told me to relax. He finally got somebody to help me out. A few days after that I quit.

There was one time I was managing the football team and I was in charge of keeping stats. I really felt out of place. Everything was surreal, in slow motion. It didn't seem real. When the team scored I was quiet, and at halftime the math teacher came up to me. He was worried that I didn't look too well. One of the guys on the team said, "What's wrong with Buddy? He looks weird." I was in denial.

These were the first episodes. I wasn't going to school for a while. I stayed home for weeks and would not go out. My mother tried to get me help. Finally I had a bad panic attack. It felt like my skin was mushy, like I had extra fat, and my legs felt very heavy when I walked. So I was rushed to the ER. Then I went to a psychiatrist the hospital recommended. They said I had Attention Deficit Disorder. I was getting a lot of different diagnoses.

BEN: I was hospitalized when I was a junior in college. In my case it came on very sudden. It didn't build up. It just happened. I remember my perception of situations, perception of just everything happening around me. At the time it seemed right to me, but to everyone else it seemed like I was acting in a bizarre way. At the time I thought there was nothing wrong with me, but with the other people.

It built up in a very short period of time and I got hospitalized. I remember every little thing I did that was bizarre. Mentally I could feel it too. My mind was not together. It was actually like muscles in my brain were having spasms. I could actually feel it in my brain. I cried at least ten times that night when I was admitted. I didn't know what was happening. Every part of my brain wasn't working. My judgment wasn't working. What other people meant when they talked I would think meant something totally different. When my parents told me, "You are wrong, you are sick, you need to get help," I didn't believe that they were saying it because they wanted to help me.

I thought they were saying it because that whole night I was having this thought that some girl was in love with me. I thought she was in the house somewhere and I went all over the house looking for her. I thought my parents were hiding her. My mind just didn't function like a normal person's.

SCHIZOPHRENIA OR PSYCHOSIS?

It is important to be aware of the distinction between psychosis and schizophrenia. *Psychosis* is a general term used to describe psychotic symptoms. Schizophrenia is a kind of psychosis. Psychotic symptoms can include:

- confusion
- inability to think clearly
- difficulty putting thoughts together
- rapid thoughts that are hard to follow
- inability to pay attention or concentrate
- confused speech

- disorganized behavior
- hallucinations such as hearing voices, seeing visions, feeling like you are being touched, smelling foul odors—all in the absence of actual stimuli

58

- extreme fear caused by the strong belief that your life is in danger even though there is no reason for such a belief.

Several brain disorders can lead to psychotic symptoms, including lesions in the brain resulting from head traumas, strokes, tumors, infections, or the use of illegal drugs. If a serious depression goes untreated for a long time, psychotic symptoms may emerge. Elderly people with dementia may develop psychosis. People with bipolar disorder (also known as manic-depressive disorder) may become psychotic. These examples show that psychosis is not necessarily the same thing as schizophrenia.

ILAN: Nobody wanted to tell me what was wrong with me, but if I didn't know what was wrong, if I didn't know the diagnosis in layman's terms, then I couldn't help stop it, help fight it, help treat it in my daily life. I was asking all around and I was getting blown off: "What do you mean, schizophrenia?" "What do you mean, nervous breakdown?" "What do you mean, I'm psychotic?" Why can't the doctors tell if you have manic depression rather than schizophrenia? Why was I thinking this way?

MAKING A DIAGNOSIS

Before doctors can arrive at a diagnosis of schizophrenia, they must make a thorough psychiatric evaluation. This includes a medical evaluation, a physical exam, a mental status exam, and appropriate tests. Some of the tests the doctors may recommend include the following:

- MRI (magnetic resonance imaging)—pictures of the brain made with special magnets to check for tumors or other structural brain changes
- CAT or CT scan (computed axial tomography)—pictures of the brain using special x-ray techniques to check for some unusual change such as a tumor
- EEG (electroencephalogram)—checking brain waves to check for seizures
- drug screening—testing the blood to make certain symptoms are

not caused by a chemical substance

- blood tests—to be sure there is not an unusual viral, bacterial, or other illness that shows up in the blood that may be causing symptoms.

Also, a full history of the illness is taken that includes any changes in thinking, behavior, movement, mood, or sensory perceptions noticed by you or by family or friends.

Other diagnoses must be excluded. Remember, there are other psychotic disorders—bipolar disorder, major depression, substance abuse, and other medical illnesses—that share many of the same symptoms; these possibilities must be eliminated before doctors will diagnose schizophrenia or schizoaffective disorder.

To make a diagnosis of schizophrenia once other illnesses are ruled out, the doctor will be looking for psychotic symptoms and significant social or school/work problems. The doctor will also be checking how long the problem has been going on. For a diagnosis of schizophrenia there must be at least six months of *some* negative symptoms and/or positive symptoms. In addition, within those six months, there must be at least one month of positive symptoms or negative symptoms for most of a month (see chapter 4). This sounds complicated, and that is probably good because it means the doctor must consider your illness very carefully to make a diagnosis.

There are also special types of schizophrenia, which are called subclassifications.

TYPES OF SCHIZOPHRENIA
Subclassifications of Schizophrenia
paranoid type—frequent auditory hallucinations or one or more delusions

disorganized type—disorganized speech and behavior, and flat or inappropriate affect

catatonic type—extreme motor immobility; purposeless, excessive motor activity; inappropriate physical postures; and repeating words or behaviors

undifferentiated type—meets criteria for the general category of schizophrenia but does not fall into any of the other types

residual type—one or more episodes of schizophrenia have occurred in the past but the current illness is essentially negative symptoms and mild positive symptoms.

Schizophreniform Disorder

Schizophreniform disorder is an illness that meets all the diagnostic requirements for schizophrenia except for duration of the symptoms displayed. In other words, if there have been symptoms for more than one month but less than six months, then a schizophreniform disorder diagnosis is made. If symptoms last more than six months, then a diagnosis of schizophrenia is made.

Schizoaffective Disorder

Like other psychotic disorders, schizoaffective disorder can be a difficult diagnosis to determine. The person must meet all the criteria for schizophrenia and have significant mood symptoms. It must then be determined that the mood symptoms are not causing the psychotic symptoms. To do this the doctor takes a careful history to know whether there have been psychotic symptoms even when there have been no mood symptoms.

DOES HENRY HAVE SCHIZOAFFECTIVE DISORDER OR SCHIZOPHRENIA OR BIPOLAR DISORDER?

Henry thought the CIA was watching him and that someone had poisoned his food. Henry said his thoughts were going very fast and that he thought he had a special relationship with God. He was filled with energy and stayed up praying for two days. That is when his girlfriend brought him to the hospital. In the hospital all his tests came back negative. There were no drugs in his system and nothing was physically wrong with Henry.

When questioned, Henry and his girlfriend told the doctors he had been thinking people were watching him since last Christmas, nearly eight months earlier. He'd stopped going to work and was sleeping during the days instead of the nights until the past weekend. He said he was not really depressed but had been very frightened and anxious for the past few months. His girlfriend said he looked depressed because he would not leave the house. Then the past weekend he'd started to have manic symptoms (not needing sleep, high energy, racing thoughts, and grandiose thinking).

At this point the doctor had a very hard time deciding whether this was bipolar disorder or schizoaffective disorder, or possibly even major depression with psychotic symptoms. Over the next six months there were often times when Henry had manic symptoms: he thought God was talking especially to him and he had a lot of sexual energy. He was also very paranoid. Then there were three or four weeks when Henry had no manic symptoms or symptoms of depression but he was very paranoid. Now the diagnosis was much clearer. The doctor told Henry he had schizoaffective disorder. The doctor made the diagnosis of schizoaffective disorder because there were periods when Henry had a mixture of psychotic and manic symptoms but he *also* experienced a period of over two weeks when he was not having any mood symptoms, only psychotic symptoms.

Schizophrenia Versus Mood Disorders

Bipolar disorder is often confused with schizophrenia or schizoaffective disorder, but it is not the same illness. It is a mood disorder characterized by manic, depressed, or mixed mood states. Symptoms of mania include elevated or irritable mood, grandiosity, decreased need for sleep, racing thoughts, distractibility, agitation, poor impulse control, and pressured speech. Depressive symptoms include sad mood, guilty feelings, poor appetite, and weight change. A mixed state has characteristics of both manic and depressed states at the same time.

The difference between bipolar disorder and schizoaffective disorder is that in bipolar disorder the mood is the main symptom. When the mood symptoms are gone the person returns to normal functioning. Similarly, in depression with psychotic symptoms, there are psychotic symptoms along with the depressed mood, and when the mood symptoms lift, the person returns to normal. In schizoaffective disorder, the mood symptoms may clear, but other symptoms continue.

Childhood-Onset Schizophrenia

Although most people who develop schizophrenia are in their late teens to mid-twenties, schizophrenia can begin at very young ages as well as much older ages. When we talk about childhood-onset schizophrenia we usually mean schizophrenia that starts before a child turns 13 years old. It is estimated that one child in 35,000 to 50,000 has schizophrenia, while the rate is one person in 100 for the general population. In other words, schizophrenia that begins before the teenage years is quite rare. Schizophrenia symptoms are the same in children as in adults, but childhood schizophrenia may be more difficult to diagnose and treat.

62   Children with schizophrenia often experience the same positive, negative, and cognitive symptoms discussed earlier in this chapter. They may hear voices, see things that are not there, feel things on their skin, or smell or taste strange things. They may feel confused, be frightened by delusions, lose their ability to attend to simple activities such as bathing and dressing, and have difficulties socializing with friends. As with other people struggling with schizophrenia, their hallucinations and delusions are based on their experiences of the world. This means that children will have psychotic experiences that are based on the television, movies, games, people, and places that they encounter. Cognitively, children with schizophrenia often have difficulty with memory and concentration required for learning. They may also have difficulties expressing thoughts and understanding what is said to them.

Although the symptoms of schizophrenia are very much the same as for all other people with schizophrenia, it is important to recognize that the symptoms are happening to children whose bodies are growing and changing every minute. Children's brains mature in complex ways that allow them to take on new social, educational, and emotional challenges. They make new friends, learn new skills, and begin to learn about who they are in relation to the world. Schizophrenia disrupts this process so that is very difficult to mature socially, emotionally, and behaviorally.

Children with schizophrenia may also have additional psychological problems. In the same way as older people, they may also have other disorders such as obsessive compulsive disorder, anxiety disorders, and mood disorders. Some children with schizophrenia also have pervasive developmental disorder (PDD). Children are said to have PDD when they have delays that show up early in development, usually by age three or four. They may have difficulties relating to friends, communicating, or imagination. They may do things like flap their hands, say things over and over, or get stuck doing something over and over. Some children with PDD also experience hallucinations now and again, making it very difficult to tell whether a child's symptoms are due to PDD or schizophrenia. Since both PDD and schizophrenia may lead to delays in development and psychosis, the diagnosis of schizophrenia may be added if a child has psychotic symptoms that continue over many months, occur in all areas of life (school, friends, and home), and affect functioning so that the child is unable to do the usual things expected for a person his or her age. As with adults and teenagers, it often takes time to tell exactly what is going on when children are having problems with thinking, feeling, and behavior.

Additional information regarding diagnosing schizophrenia:

NIMH:

http://www.nimh.nih.gov/health/publications/schizophrenia/index.shtml.

You can also order a copy of the publication (English or Spanish).

NAMI: www.nami.org. Follow the link to "schizophrenia."

Diagnostic and Statistical Manual of Mental Disorders: DSM-IV (American Psychiatric Association, 2000).

7

WHAT WILL PEOPLE THINK OF ME NOW?

It is not easy to know how people will react to your illness. There is a stigma related to schizophrenia based on common stereotypes of people with schizophrenia as frightening, dangerous, and different. Like all stereotypes, these are based on ignorance and generalizations.

So how do you handle the worry about what people may be thinking of you? First, think about your own preconceptions regarding people with schizophrenia. What did you think before you were sick? Most of the people writing this book had their own mistaken ideas about this illness.

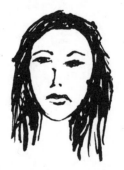

ZELDA

ZELDA: If you have to put a clear label on it, it's schizophrenia. But I don't side strongly with labels and classifications, as they try to fit things into boxes. Doctors and therapists asked me way back when if I felt comfortable with that "diagnosis," and I answered, "That's fine."

ILAN: I think the biggest problem in the beginning was admitting to old friends, even old friends I knew I could trust, what was wrong. I wouldn't tell anybody that I had a mental illness and that I had spent time in a mental hospital.

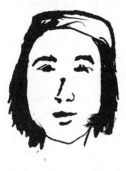

ILAN

I had recently returned from a year of study in Israel. I started school and had a very successful semester. I was on a high until I lost a peer I had known from elementary school. Over the summer I lost two more people. I wasn't ready to tackle school again. I broke down in the emergency room completely. I woke up some time after and they said, "You had a nervous breakdown." I was in complete denial. I was sure if they let me out of the locked door I could handle myself just fine.

Some time thereafter my father took me for a haircut and I still couldn't pull myself together. I needed my father to do a lot of the talking. After my first visit home I realized that something was very wrong. I spent the day in bed. I couldn't sit long enough to eat a bowl of cornflakes. I thought I could spend time with my grandmother, who was a favorite of mine, but I couldn't focus. I just wanted to lie down.

I don't think I had a good understanding of what schizophrenia was before I came to the hospital. The little that I knew about it was what I saw on TV. I carried with me all of the stereotypes of mental illness. One of the things I had in mind was that once you have schizophrenia you stay sick. You don't come out of the hospital for the rest of your life. I always passed Creedmore on the street when we would go somewhere. I knew it was a mental institution, and it really did look quite final, the bars on the windows and doors that you never saw anybody go into or anybody go out of. And many of the talk shows project people with schizophrenia as having multiple personalities. That misconception along with the others is what I brought with me.

66   I remember conversations with several friends who didn't know about my illness. I would tell them what happened and I would say, "Are you still my friend?" Most of the time they did stay my friends. I was looking for a job, and I would take anything I thought I might qualify for. Many of the schools would take people without licenses [as teachers]. So I went to this private school and the man was very happy with my credentials. But once I told him that I have schizophrenia, that was it. I called and called. So I just can't tell anybody if I want the job. I would be careful whom you tell what kind of insurance you have, because people will know that if you have this kind of insurance you are disabled. Especially if the illness is invisible, you don't need to share it with anybody, especially at a job. You want to get by looking as normal as possible. The whole world carries within them the stigma of schizophrenia and they will stigmatize you. People who have a stigma didn't put it on themselves. It was put on them.

MYTHS, LABELS, AND STEREOTYPES

The stigma of schizophrenia makes it difficult for those with the illness to live openly, to get support, or to apply for school or work. Because most people do not understand schizophrenia, they think about the illness in terms of stereotypes. Common stereotypes depict people with schizophrenia as retarded, drug addicted, homeless, dangerous, crazy, evil, not "normal," bad, weak, different, or having multiple personalities. These labels are hard to live with especially because they are no more true for people with schizophrenia than for other people. In the face of these stereotypes, people with schizophrenia have a lot of questions: How can I go on with my life? How can I tell my family and friends? How can I go to school or work?

DEALING WITH PREJUDICES AND STEREOTYPES

Step 1—Learn all you can about schizophrenia.

Step 2—Put the feelings of shame behind you.

Step 3—Surround yourself with strong supports such as family, good friends, group members, counselors, and doctors.

Step 4—Decide for yourself whom you want to tell (friends or family) and whom you need to tell (doctors, school administrators, and employers).

Step 5—Work toward staying well.

Remember, you are not schizophrenic! This is not an identity. You have a disease called schizophrenia.

LUCINDA: Before I got sick I thought schizophrenia was a change in personality, multiple personalities. I know I read it somewhere. I wonder why so many people think it's that? I heard it or read it somewhere. I didn't come to the conclusion that schizophrenia is multiple personality disorder on my own.

LAURIE: I didn't have any idea schizophrenia existed. I just thought retarded people were the only ones who got sick. I used to be afraid of them, that they would hurt me. I feel safer now that I know what is going on.

BUDDY: I thought schizophrenia was a disorder where a person would have multiple, split personalities, like five or ten different personalities. I was completely wrong about that.

GENEVIVE: At first I thought schizophrenia referred to people with split personalities or people who were catatonic, in a state where they can't talk. I thought you had to do something that is destructive to be mentally ill. Before my brother got sick I thought it was a homeless person's illness, being on drugs. But then when my brother got sick I realized it's not just people out on the street. It happens to normal people. My brother jumped out the window to try to kill himself. People get sick. It's just that I have this illness. My brother is mentally ill, so I know now that it could be hereditary. And my sister was ill. She saw a psychiatrist for a while and then she stopped.

AUDREY: I think I used to think schizophrenia meant a split personality because of the Greek or Latin root of the word. It means "split mind." Actually it doesn't mean split mind, but it translates that way.

JOSEPH: I think a huge misconception about mental illness is in the labeling. When somebody says they have schizophrenia or they are manic-depressive, people in general think they are the most evil people to exist. But if you think about it, people who have mental illness can accomplish just as much as, if not more than, a "normal" person, because I honestly believe that nobody is truly, absolutely normal.

GARY: Before I got sick I thought schizophrenia meant, vaguely, a crazy person. I was never aware that this was a legitimate physical illness.

BEN: I didn't know about schizophrenia. I learned in health class people usually think schizophrenia is split personality, but it's not. That's all I remember.

LUCINDA: Of course there is a stigma. People just think you are crazy and you are somebody they shouldn't get to know because of fear. They just fear for themselves that you might turn around and do something. I know even myself, before I was diagnosed, I would look at a person with mental illness as different. I probably wouldn't want to know them. I would be afraid of them because they are just not all there. Now I think differently. I think it could happen to anybody, anytime. I think of people with mental illness as the same as anybody else.

STIGMA AND SCHIZOPHRENIA

AUDREY: In the beginning I was very confused. I knew something was wrong, but I couldn't answer the questions and I was ashamed at what was happening. It was very scary and I felt very alone. I felt that I was the only person on earth with the problems I had. And I hid it so that it was even harder for anyone to figure out what it was. I became more and more depressed and finally became so depressed that I was psychotic. I didn't eat. I lost my appetite. I think it was my way of showing outwardly that I was in pain. I got to the point where my mother had to dress me, bathe me, put clothes on me, and help me to eat. It wasn't until then that my parents had to own up to the fact that I was sick. Out of desperation they took me to the hospital.

BEN: Stigma and any type of bias or stereotype stem from lack of knowledge. When people don't know enough about these illnesses, they think all these bad things. I am from an Asian family. They view mental illness as cancer. They shun the whole idea. They just deny. "That can't be happening to my kids." Asian families take it harder. They are not as liberal. Asian people think of people with mental illness as killers. A lot of stuff doesn't make sense, but that bad people thing is attached to mental illness. It's not true.

PATRICK: When I first got sick I thought schizophrenia was just a name with a lot of letters in it. Society thinks that anybody who has it is crazy. People don't want to talk about it. They feel ashamed of it. Once in a while I feel that way, but being around people and being on the medication lift the cloud.

GARY: Stigma plays a big part in my life. Because of the stigma I am always concealing my illness. I had a good two years removed from my life. There is a gap in my employment and school history I am always thinking how to cover up. Sometimes I have to lie and say that I have been working, say that I took a few semesters off. I won't say why, just that I didn't know what I wanted to do and took a few years off. Only four of my closest friends know I had the illness, and sometimes I don't even tell them about seeing my therapist and psychiatrist. I know they'll accept me, but that's how powerful the stigma of schizophrenia is. When people think about schizophrenia they don't think it's a serious illness like cancer or AIDS. They think that people are just crazy. I don't blame them; I used to think the same. As a result of the stigma I can't be open about my life.

JAMES: When I got out of the hospital I saw a couple of shows and the way they hyped up schizophrenia wasn't half of what I had seen. But they showed people who were criminals. There was one that I saw that I related to in the movies. The hype is true in a way. It has to be true because there are hospitals and institutions researching the problem of schizophrenia. I am not a criminal, a bad guy. I met a lot of people that are real good. Everybody I've met in this hospital is really nice.

WHOM TO TELL

It can be very frightening to think about looking for a job and having to disclose information about your illness to potential employers. The law regarding disclosure is a federal law (Americans with Disabilities Act), which means it applies to all fifty states plus Puerto Rico.

As a rule, employers are not allowed to ask you if you have a history of mental illness when you apply for a job. There are some special jobs, such as law enforcement and armed service positions, where employers are allowed to ask about psychiatric illnesses and medications. In those cases they must ask every applicant. If a physical or psychiatric test is required for the job, it must be given to everyone applying for it and jobs similar to it. Employers may ask you about substance abuse, but not about legitimate use of prescription drugs.

Once you are hired you may disclose your illness in order to get what are known as reasonable accommodations. These include a flexible sched-

69

ule so you can see your doctor or counselor, a special office setup to help with your concentration, and even a job coach if you need one. *You may not be fired* for making this disclosure, although employers do have the right to ask for evidence of your disability in writing. Employers must keep documentation of your illness in separate, confidential files, and they may not allow this information to become known to your fellow workers. Remember, if you need special accommodations because of your illness, you must ask for them through your supervisor or the personnel department.

Schools also must provide reasonable accommodations and may not ask you about your illness when you apply. Again, to get accommodations you must ask for them, usually through the Dean of Students. All of these rights are part of a recent ruling based on the Americans with Disabilities Act of 1990. If you think you have been treated unfairly, contact the Equal Employment Opportunity Commission at 1–800–669–4000 or tell your counselor. There also may be state laws that protect you. Usually the phone numbers for state offices are found in the state government section of your phone book.

AUDREY: It takes some strength and some time to completely recover. I found that it was very difficult for me to function in social situations. I felt as though I were walking around with two heads. And that everybody knew that I was crazy. The hardest thing that I experienced in high school was that because my friends could not handle my being sick, they abandoned me. Now I was completely alone and felt extremely alienated.

My peers stigmatized me in high school to the extent that I was completely outcast. I had never been so hurt. That year I felt so alienated by my classmates that I moved in with relatives out west and graduated from high school there. I was admitted to college out there with a scholarship. From my experience I've learned that the illness is only a small part of who I am, and it is not necessary to inform everyone about it.

SAMANTHA: I'm still so new with dealing with the stigma that when I apply for and get jobs and go to work I don't know if I should tell them I have a mental illness. I'm nervous because I'm expected to do the same job as any other person. There is stigma to worry about when I go to dance classes and I'm making friends and people want to know why my daughter is not living with me. I don't say very much about it because of the stigma and misunderstanding people have about it. So I really haven't been very open outside my family about it.

ZELDA: The word *schizophrenic* definitely carries a stigma. I really haven't had firsthand experience, but I know I don't share that with everyone I know. Like, my boss doesn't have any idea that happened. If I had asthma or something of that nature, it wouldn't be a big deal. Before I got sick I thought this disease was multiple personality disorder. I saw *Sybil* and thought she had schizophrenia.

71

BETH: All my friends and family were very supportive. My friends were shocked. The guy I was dating said, "Whoa." He didn't know what to think. But when I went back to school they all knew about mental illness. I wound up giving a speech in my class. Nobody looked at me differently at all. I think everybody was very cool with it. I never lost any friends. But I'm afraid to tell people. I hear all the time people making fun of crazy people, and I say, "You don't know what you are talking about." That bothers me. Because of the stigma I just tell people I am close with and people I need to tell. In my field I probably could tell people because they know about schizophrenia. But I don't tell them; it's just better, unless something happened and my symptoms started.

JOSEPH: To tell a new friend, somebody I just met, I feel a little embarrassed, stressed a little. But when I think about it there is nothing really to be embarrassed about. If the person can't understand that I had an episode, then he's not my friend. Try to keep it to yourself as much as possible. If you feel someone should know because it is a part of you and you really want that person to know you, by all means tell him. If you don't feel someone should know, a job, acquaintance, by all means don't tell.

JACKIE: I was a little worried about the stigma, so I only told a few close friends. My mother had told the whole family. I realized that nobody treated me differently. My aunt didn't want to face it and didn't want to talk about it, but I didn't have any problems.

Usually when I tell people what I have I explain to them what it is. When I tell people about my schizophrenia I don't just tell them that I have schizophrenia. I tell them what it is because most people don't know. Tell only close friends. I don't feel it's necessary to tell employers. I told my boyfriends.

ROMAN: My band member is bipolar. He told me, "I have a whole bunch of schizophrenic friends, don't I." I tell only certain people—my close friends, that's about it. For the job I won't tell them about the illness.

It's not a real stressful job. They might think that because I have a disability I might not be able to perform the job.

MIKE: I was concerned that people would look at me differently. But nobody really treated me differently. They were still nice, cool. My friends stayed the same. I would recommend that people tell their family, definitely doctors, social workers, people who can really help you.

I wouldn't recommend telling your friends right away because you don't know what type of response you are going to get and you want people who are really going to support you. Relatives, close people. That's about it. I would just go for a job; I wouldn't mention my disability. As far as school, I would let them know because this has to do with my mind and concentration. I would let them know so they could provide whatever they could to help me. And I know that they have programs at the college I applied to, so I would recommend telling your school.

GENEVIVE: I was afraid to let people know I have schizophrenia. I thought, this is not something that you talk about and tell friends, because people are going to treat you differently, look at you differently. They are going to think you are going to do something bad. Especially because on TV when somebody commits a crime, they often say that the person is mentally ill. People think when you are mentally ill you are going to do something bad. If you want to discuss it, wait until you are well and good so you can really convince the person you are not what society thinks you are. Wait until you get better. Then you can explain to people if you want to. Only my family knows.

After I got out of the hospital, that's when my mother told a couple of her friends. It was okay because they are close friends. I knew they knew about my brother and they knew I wasn't going to commit a crime. At first, when I was still having symptoms, I didn't want her to tell anyone. No friends of mine know I am mentally ill. At first I didn't want people to know, but my counselor told me to go to the disabilities counselors in the college. I got tutoring. I have a counselor to talk to if I have a problem and they help me with choosing my classes. I get first choice of classes. I get to have extra time taking my test. I don't know how I would do if I didn't have that program.

BUDDY: I don't really tell people that I have schizophrenia, that I see a psychiatrist, or that I have a social worker. I'm afraid they might see me in a different light, like I'm crazy or something. I haven't told my girlfriend. I told her I was depressed in high school. I think she would understand because her best friend's mother has schizophrenia. I've only told the friends who came to see me in the hospital, and they don't know what I have. I keep it confidential, and I don't think it is really important for them to know, unless they see changes in my behavior, which I really doubt. I don't think you should tell any job because I think it might ruin your chances. The employer who is doing the interview might not have an understanding of the disease schizophrenia and he might be ignorant. He might not want to give you the opportunity because he is afraid of that word.

JAMES: I think you should tell your boss, your immediate family, and your friends. You tell them certain symptoms so they'll tell you if they notice you are getting sick again. Don't tell anybody when you first meet. The other person will think they have to deal with you and your problem. A couple of times I did and they never really asked me any questions about it. A few females I told, but then the relationship didn't go too far. I told one guy in a joking way. He joked about it, "Well, now we have another crazy person employed here with us."

SHARON: My sister always teases me. When I speak to her she tells me I'm lucky because I have Medicaid. Some people treat you differently. They don't act the same with you. They single you out from everybody else. I don't know what they think. I think they would rather not be bothered because they don't understand. I remember when I went to church while I was still very medicated. I went to the bathroom and they were looking at me funny. They think God can cure you, can take it away from you.

ABBY: I don't mind explaining to someone in my group or the doctors about my illness, but it depends on who. People might not think you are in your right mind, and fewer people will talk to you. If I were to go somewhere socializing and I were to say, "Excuse me, I have a mental illness," they would say, "She is not right." They might think I need to be in the hospital. I try to avoid telling people. I don't tell people I am in the day program. People might treat you differently; they might not even know how to act. They might say to themselves, "I have to be careful." They might think you are a very weak person.

JEFF: You shouldn't tell the people you work with. I found that out. They label you as a nut job. They tease you. They treat it like it's a joke when it really isn't. It's really pretty serious. You should tell your family, people you are close to. People like that you can tell. I told one friend, but he was

73

scared to visit me. People have bad stereotypes. My brother's friends came by, and that was nice that they visited me.

ALEXIS: I feel people should be more educated about the illness before they make judgments. You have to be selective whom you tell, because a lot of people will judge you even if you are capable of doing a good job. People are ignorant and people can be cruel. Even if they have known you for many years as a highly functional person and would never guess that you had any mental illness, if they did find out they could, unfortunately, change their opinion of you. For example, I told my boyfriend only because we had the intention of getting married. Otherwise I wouldn't have been so free to give the information away. I was scared about telling him because I thought there was a good chance he would break up with me. I was prepared to deal with it. But he was very accepting and understanding. He had a lot of questions, but he still wants to marry me, and even though he knows it's hereditary he still wants to have a family.

When I did tell him I felt like an anchor had been lifted and there were no more secrets. I couldn't lead a life with him hiding that. Sooner or later he would have found out, and that could have caused a divorce or something terrible. Still, I'm ashamed to tell my boyfriend about the hospital because people stigmatize. I feel maybe it's worse if someone goes into the hospital. When people hear about a psychiatric hospital they think you're off the wall, violent. At my first hospital people were violent. I was scared there. I am afraid he will think of me as very sick, in a very unstable light if I tell him about the hospital.

BUCK: Nobody knows I am sick. Only my family knows because I think people would look at me in a different way. Like some sort of crazy person, like any minute I could go and do something out of the normal. Maybe fight. Something in my mind would click and I would do something bad.

VAN: I'd be very careful whom you tell what happened. Make sure you tell family members you trust and only friends you really trust. Don't let anyone know you are on medication.

ALEXANDRA: My family knows and so does my boyfriend. I think you should tell your parents about your illness and your friends if they ask you what happened. I won't just tell anybody because I think they might look at you different.

VANESSA: The only one I speak to about it is my oldest sister, because she went through something similar. She stopped her medication, but she wouldn't tell me to stop. She says if anything happens she would call her doctor and start all over again. I don't talk to anybody about it because I don't think they would understand. Some of my friends have asked me to explain it to them, to explain what happened, but I don't think they would understand. I think they would laugh if I told them half the stuff that I've been through. It's not funny. It's painful. It's really scary.

MARCUS: I don't want people to see me differently. If I tell them I have a mental illness they might see me differently, like not want to hang out with me. I don't really tell my friends. They might see me differently. "We better not hang out with him because he's sick." I tell my family and doctors because they can help. I just tell employers I had a sickness. I don't tell them what I had.

AMBER: My family knows that I have schizophrenia. I told my best friend I was in the hospital, that I was very confused but now I am getting well, and that I am going on with my life. I guess I'm still a little worried about the stigma of the illness. I guess I don't want them to think I have multiple personalities or say, "Oh my god, she has schizophrenia, that must be bad." I don't want them to look at me in that way. I don't think I would tell employers because I still care what other people think about me. I know at times I shouldn't, but I think I would feel better if they didn't know about it.

BEAUX: I feel like people, family, friends label you. Everybody loves you, but there's still a little bit of that label on you. I try not to let it bother me. Whatever I do, I try to put my energy into it. I'm not sitting around thinking about it because that's not good. I try not to tell friends. My job knows. I would have preferred for them not to know because of the labeling.

MEREDITH: Discuss with family whom to tell. I don't think right away you should tell anybody. But as time goes on you can. It takes time to accept it in your life. It takes time for other people to accept it.

SAM: I believe people will shun me if I tell them. Like if I want to go out with a girl, I am sure there will be a change in her dealings with me. But if I said I have asthma or diabetes?

THOMAS: I think you shouldn't hide it. Tell your family, but if someone else finds out it depends on who it is. I would tell people if I went for a job.

SAMANTHA: I have a little girl, and my daughter knows that something has been wrong with me for a long time. Exactly what, I haven't explained yet because she is pretty young and wouldn't understand. I don't want to cause her any more extra stress than she is probably experiencing because of our separation.

You have to tell your mom and dad. You have to tell the apartment program; your social worker, your doctor, the medical center where you are getting your care have to know what is happening. You have to use your discretion in what you say to people and whom you trust with this information.

BEN: Some family members are blabbermouths. Obviously immediate family should be the ones you tell because this type of illness affects you negatively. If you want to get a job, that will affect you. And people look at you differently if you tell them you have schizophrenia. People in your classes won't want to sit next to you.

This issue of whom you should tell conflicts a little with what counselors tell you, that you shouldn't be afraid or ashamed. Basically, no one should know. Don't feel bad you have it, but we live in a world that's not all nice people.

RICHIE: I tell some people, but when I meet a new girl I pretend I don't have anything wrong with me. When you trust a person that you know, like after you know them for a while. . . . I don't say anything when I go for a job because a lot of people fear what they don't understand. The people I told didn't make fun of me, so I had good experiences.

ZELDA: I think you should tell anyone that's close to you, and hopefully they will accept it. At first I would hold back from any school you are trying to get into or any job you are trying to get. It's not a casual mention, like "I had chicken pox and I had schizophrenia."

> There are no rules about whom to tell. Each person makes up his or her own mind about telling friends and family members. The people you *must* tell are your doctors and therapists.

For more information about stigma and schizophrenia:

NAMI's StigmaBusters. See the Web site for the National Alliance for the Mentally Ill, www.nami.org, and click on their link to "stigma."

MentalHelp.net: www.mentalhelp.net/. Enter "schizophrenia and stigma" in the search box to get the latest article.

Mental Health America: www.nmha.org/

Me, Myself, and Them: A Firsthand Account of One Young Person's Experience with Schizophrenia, by Kurt Snyder, Raquel E. Gur, and Linda Wasmer Andrews (Oxford University Press, 2007).

8 MEDICATION

A lot of people dislike taking medicine for a lot of different reasons. Medications often have side effects: they can make some people gain weight, drool, or feel tired, strange, or stiff. Other people do not want to take any kind of medicine because of their religious or health beliefs. Still others feel they should be strong enough to control the symptoms themselves without any kind of help.

Nevertheless, medicine is absolutely necessary for a return to health. For this reason it is important to become familiar with medicines, how they work, and the problems they may cause.

I HATE PILLS

BUCK: I was twenty-two when I got sick. That was three years ago. The first time I got sick I didn't know what was wrong. I was feeling paranoid and I didn't know what to do. I knew it was something, but I didn't know I had schizophrenia. I stayed at home, couldn't go out. I felt like people were watching me. I was hearing voices. Then my mom sent me to a clinic on Long Island, and I was telling the doctor what happened. The doctor gave me medicine. I was still feeling the same way, so they sent me into the hospital. That was the first time I had ever been to a mental institution.

The doctors were asking what was wrong with me, and I told them I was hearing voices. I had this feeling that something was crawling on my

Special contributor: Julia Becker, M.D.

body. I was having hallucinations, like seeing things that weren't there, this person with red eyes I thought was God. When they admitted me they gave me a shot to calm me down. The next day I was feeling a little better, but then I was feeling stiff, like I couldn't walk. Something was wrong with my right side. I thought the right side of my body was fighting the other side. I couldn't walk that well. After a few days I was feeling better.

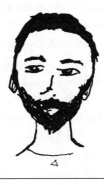

BUCK

After a couple of months I went home and attended the day program. It was going pretty good. I used to go to all of my groups. Then I was taking my medication steadily. After a couple of months I stopped taking my medication, and I got sick again. I started to think people were following me. I started hearing voices again, and I ended up back in the hospital. The doctor told me that I was diagnosed with schizophrenia and that it was a mental illness. That's when I realized that something had been wrong with my mind. So I finally recognized that it was something in my mind I could not control. It was very scary.

The third time I went into the hospital the same thing happened. That's when I finally realized I had to take the medication.

I hate the feeling that pills give me. Medication makes me tired, sleepy. Makes me feel I don't want to do anything. Makes me gain weight. Sometimes it makes me nauseated. It's just the whole idea of taking pills turns me off. I hate waking up knowing I have to take pills in the morning and at night. I hate taking pills because I think I don't need them. I thought the problem was something in my mind that I could control without taking anything. When I was growing up my family told me that you don't have to take medicine. None of my family used to take pills. I didn't even know there were pills for such things as schizophrenia.

MEREDITH: It makes you feel sicker the more you take. People complain about taking Tylenol. I pop seven pills every night.

ROMAN: The pills make me sleepy and they make me sleep late. At the beginning there are a lot of side effects—I broke out in rashes on my arms and chest. Weight gain—it makes you eat a lot.

I really don't want to stay on the medication, but I have to. I went off my medication for three months—I couldn't get the blood tests anymore because I couldn't get to the lab. I was working. Three months later I started to get sick again. I was hearing voices. I was getting emotional messages—I'd watch TV and then I would concentrate on one thing and constantly think about that one thing. I called the doctor and I came in. She put me on a different medication so I wouldn't be getting blood tests every week. That was the only time I stopped.

GARY: In the hospital I didn't want to take pills because I thought they were trying to give me illegal substances to make me stay there longer. Later it was the side effects I didn't like.

ZELDA: I feel like I am on a leash. It dictates to me when I should go to sleep and how much rest I'll need in order to wake up on time. And no drinking at all. Getting used to having a needle in my arm every week is something I would never do. Now it's every other week.

ANTIPSYCHOTIC MEDICINES AND SCHIZOPHRENIA

At this point there is no cure for schizophrenia, but it is treatable with medication and therapy. Medications are necessary to manage symptoms and to improve your ability to enjoy life. Technology is developing rapidly, and hope exists for improved medications and, possibly, a cure for schizophrenia.

Antipsychotic medications are used to treat psychotic symptoms in schizophrenia as well as in other psychotic disorders of the brain. These medications have been available since the 1950s. The first medication ever used, in 1950, was Chlorpromazine (thorazine). Since then many others have been developed. Within just the past few years there have been a number of new ones put on the market, and others are in the process of being tested.

The precise mechanism by which antipsychotic medicine works is unknown. This is a major area of current research. One belief is that psychotic symptoms are related to overactivity in the brain of the neurotransmitter dopamine. It is thought that antipsychotic medications reduce the activity of dopamine in the synaptic cleft (see figure 3.5 on page 35). They do this by blocking the dopamine receptors—that is, by preventing dopamine from attaching to the receptors. These medications may also affect several other neurotransmitters in the brain, such as serotonin, norepinephrine, and glutamate. The overall purpose of antipsychotic treatment is to restore the disturbed chemical balance of the brain.

81

Different medications affect different receptors and, because everyone is unique, they affect each person differently. People may need different doses of the same medicine, and some may respond better to certain medicines than to others.

Too much dopamine activity may be the cause of symptoms. Some medicines act as blockers. They stop dopamine from getting through to the receiving neuron.

First-Generation Medications

Since 1950, many antipsychotic medications have been developed. The first-generation group is called the *typical* or *conventional* medications. There are many first-generation antipsychotic medications. Some of the more popularly used include Haldol (haloperidol), Prolixin (fluphenazine), Navane (thiothixene), Trilafon (perphenazine), and Moban (molindone). Haldol and Prolixin can be given by injection, like an antibiotic shot, one to two times a month, instead of orally. Some common side effects of "typical" medications like Haldol and Prolixin include prolonged but reversible muscle stiffness; muscle cramping of the neck, fingers, or eyes; tremors; dry mouth; weight gain; and tardive dyskinesia (involuntary muscle movements). Tardive dyskinesia may be permanent despite discontinuation of the medication. The risk of tardive dyskinesia is 4 percent per year of exposure to typical antipsychotic medications. The doctor will regularly do exams to check for this side effect.

Second-Generation Medications

More recently, a new generation of medications sometimes called *atypical* (not typical) antipsychotics has become available. These were designed to have fewer side effects and appear to be more effective at treating the negative symptoms of schizophrenia. The risk of tardive dyskinesia associated with atypical antipsychotics is lower than with typical antipsychotics.

Weight gain is a significant side effect of several of these newer medications. Related to this weight gain is an important health issue called metabolic syndrome. Metabolic syndrome is a group of conditions that include increased insulin levels, excess fat around the waist area, high cholesterol levels, and elevated blood pressure. Together these health problems increase the risk of heart disease, stroke, and diabetes. Although it is less likely, it is possible that even without weight gain these medications may put you at higher risk for diabetes and elevated cholesterol.

Be sure to have a checkup every six months with your medical doctor to make certain you are not developing metabolic syndrome. Also, be aware of the warning signs of diabetes and get checked immediately if you are experiencing possible symptoms.

The warning signs of diabetes are as follows:

- urinating a lot more than usual
- being very thirsty
- losing weight without reason
- feeling exceptionally tired
- patches of velvety dark, thick skin under your arms.

See chapter 9's section on healthy eating and staying active to help prevent metabolic syndrome.

Some notes about side effects: All antipsychotic medications can cause NMS (neuroleptic malignant syndrome). NMS is very rare, but if you develop the symptoms—high fever, stiff muscles, and confusion—you must get medical help quickly. All medicines can cause sexual side effects, restlessness, and a variety of other problems not mentioned previously. Your doctor and pharmacist can provide additional information. All pharmaceutical companies also have Web sites with a great deal of information as well as telephone numbers you can call for more details.

Abilify (aripiprazole) is an antipsychotic medication that causes less weight gain and less tiredness for many people. It can cause a feeling of restlessness, which can make you feel quite uncomfortable, as well as muscle stiffness.

Clozaril (clozapine) was the first of the atypical medications to be introduced. Clozapine is the only antipsychotic that does not cause tardive dyskinesia at all. It also works well for people with schizophrenia that has not been very responsive to other medications. Common side effects include tremors of the arms, hands, and legs; restlessness; muscle stiffness; sedation; drooling (which usually occurs at night); weight gain; and constipation.

There is also a 1 percent chance that a person taking clozapine will develop agranulocytosis, which is a decrease in the number of infection-fighting cells in the body. This is a risky situation. Blood tests are done weekly for six months in order to watch closely for the occurrence of this side effect. If the tests have been negative, the risk of having a seriously low white cell count becomes extremely low. After the six-month period is passed successfully, blood tests are performed only once every two weeks. If all continues to go well, at twelve months blood testing is only once a month. If the cell count becomes too low, the doctor may discontinue the medication briefly, do blood tests more frequently, or consult with a hematologist. Some doctors add lithium to bring up the white blood count. If you have a sore throat or fever while taking clozapine, call your doctor.

Be extra careful to take clozapine daily because it leaves your body very quickly. Just missing a day or two can lead to a full return of symptoms.

Fanapt (iloperidone) is the newest medication at the time of this writing. The company reports possible side effects of dizziness, dry mouth, fatigue, nausea, orthostatic hypotension, tachycardia, nasal congestion, and weight gain. It may also affect heart rhythm, which you will want to discuss with your doctor.

Geodon (zaprasidone) has the benefit of low weight gain. Some common side effects are tiredness, headache, nausea, constipation, cough, and runny nose. For some people it can cause changes in heart rhythm, which you should discuss with your doctor.

Risperdal (risperidone) was the first of the atypicals that could be used without weekly blood work. It works on both the dopamine and serotonin systems of neurotransmitters. Possible side effects include weight gain, sedation, tremors, muscle stiffness, low blood pressure, dizziness, insomnia, and anxiety. Some people also develop problems with sexual functioning; females may develop breast milk and stop menstruating. *Invega (paliperidone)* is related to Risperdal. It works much the same but uses a time-release method so that the medicine is delivered over a twenty-four-hour period.

Saphris (asenapine) is an atypical antipsychotic approved for use in 2009. Possible side effects are the inability to sit still or stop moving around (akathisia), drowsiness, and decreased oral sensitivity. It is not recommended for use by elderly people with dementia.

Seroquel (quetiapine) is another new antipsychotic medication. Possible side effects include sedation, memory problems, stomach upset, and agitation. Doctors recommend that consumers taking it have special eye examinations, because an animal study showed that beagles taking high doses developed cataracts.

Zyprexa (olanzapine)'s most common side effects include sedation, weight gain, and restlessness. Muscle rigidity, muscle twitches, and stiffness are additional possible side effects.

NEW FORMS OF MEDICATION Antipsychotic medications now come in several forms. Instead of the usual pills, some medications are available as injections, liquids, or in dissolving formats. The liquid medications and medications that dissolve in your mouth can be great if you do not like swallowing pills or have had problems with taking your medication in the past. Injectable medications have been around for years, but now several of the newer medicines are also available (or will be in the near future) in injectable forms. Injectables have the advantage of lasting for several weeks. This can be a big help for people who really do not want to take pills or have a hard time remembering to take their medicine. Some doctors and consumers even think that injectables may work better than pills.

Additional Medications

Your doctor may notice that you have developed some mood symptoms, such as depression. Therefore, he or she may prescribe lithium, Tegretol (carbamazepine), or Depakote (valproic acid) to boost the response of your antipsychotic medications, or to help stabilize mood problems and impulsive, unpredictable, or violent behavior caused by the schizophrenia.

Lithium is a salt used to stabilize mood symptoms. For people taking clozapine, lithium is sometimes used to keep white blood cell counts up. If you are taking lithium, it is important during hot weather to drink enough fluids. Dehydration can lead to increased levels of lithium, which can be dangerous. Other signs that there is too much lithium in your system include stomach upset, diarrhea, severe tremors, confusion, and lethargy. Don't worry—your doctor will go over this with you. Blood tests to monitor for therapeutic levels of lithium and to monitor for any potential toxic effects on the thyroid or kidneys should be done on a regular basis.

Tegretol (carbamazepine) is an antiseizure medication that is also used to stabilize moods or impulsive behaviors. Side effects include decrease in blood cells or platelets (cells that help blood clots form). Routine blood counts and platelet level tests will be ordered, though these problems are not common. Other side effects include motor coordination problems, stomach upset, drowsiness, and, less frequently, blurry or double vision. Tegretol renders birth control pills ineffective.

Depakote (valproic acid) is another medication that stabilizes moods and treats impulsive behaviors. Some common side effects are drowsiness, stomach upset, diarrhea, and changes in liver functions and cell counts that require occasional monitoring.

Cogentin (benztropine) is a medication used to help with side effects of stiffness, restlessness, and muscle rigidity. Too much benztropine can cause a "spacey" feeling and troubled thinking. It is important to take the prescribed dose.

Inderol (propranolol) is also used to help with side effects of restlessness.

> The list of side effects is frightening, but many people experience only a few side effects, and some people have none at all. If you do experience side effects, tell your doctor so your medications can be adjusted.

There are various additional medications that may be prescribed for problems with mood, anxiety, side effects, and other symptoms. Your treatment team will be able to provide information about these.

SIDE EFFECTS ARE NO FUN

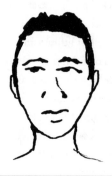

BEN

BEN: The first time at the hospital I don't remember much—at first I didn't realize where I was. When it came to me that I was at a place where they try to get mental patients to recover, it didn't bother me. What bothered me was the medication. I'm really sensitive to the antipsychotic drugs. I get so restless I can't sit still. The medicine, Prolixin and Risperdal, bothered me so much.

The first time I came out of the hospital I just stayed out of school, and I was having a problem accepting that I was sick. It hits you. Like, damn, I'm a mentally ill person. And there's a stigma. When I got home I had a problem with the medication. Again, I was too restless. I couldn't live. When I look back on it now, they gave me the wrong medicine. So I was hospitalized three or four times. But each time it had to do with the medication. I didn't take it. I would rather get sick than get the side effects.

I'm a person in unlucky circumstances who got lucky because I was surrounded by people who cared a lot. The doctors communicated very well. I think that was very important, because if you don't communicate with your doctors they don't know how you feel. You need to give them insight into yourself so they really can help you. You have to talk to them, let them know because your treatment is dependent on the doctor, and if you can really make that communication work you have a much better chance of finding a treatment that is suited to you. The chances of controlling your illness are much, much better.

JEFF: I had some problems when I took the Prolixin. It used to make me really tired and sleepy, and I almost crashed my car going to work. Now

I take olanzapine. One thing I don't like with this medicine is the weight gain. I'm trying to get rid of the weight I've gained, but it is not easy. For a while there, after the problem was over, I thought maybe I didn't need to take as much because I was not having as bad a time.

SAMANTHA: I hate it. It makes me realize that I really do have a mental illness. There are many side effects that I dislike. I've struggled with weight gain, blurry vision, caustic digestion, crabby disposition.

MIKE: I didn't know what the pills were for at first because I didn't know what was wrong with me. The side effects are just the worst—weight gain; my mind was kind of slow, I couldn't think fast enough; sleeping a lot. I couldn't take that. I felt that I could get better on my own so I didn't need the pills. I felt that if I prayed enough, God would take care of everything and I wouldn't need all this medicine. Being in denial of my whole illness was another reason I didn't want to take the pills.

SAM: I always felt clozapine was going to be a burden. And it is, with taking the blood test every two weeks. Somebody said it's not such a big deal, it's like brushing your teeth. People with AIDS take forty tablets. Three tablets are okay with me. Also, my uncle has diabetes and he takes a pill every day.

VAN: I hated the drooling, the constipation, the low libido (sex drive); and the high appetite was the worst. But I would rather spend the rest of my life out of the hospital and have no symptoms ever again. Stopping the medication affected my sleep, and that concerned me. I didn't want to have symptoms again, so I decided to continue drug treatment with a more suitable medication.

ABBY: One time I had tremors, so they gave me Cogentin. The Cogentin gave me other side effects. Also, the medicine increased my appetite and I gained weight.

MARCUS: The first time I took risperidone, and in a way it made it worse. I had the shakes in my hands, I wasn't eating, and I couldn't sleep; I still felt paranoid. It didn't help. Then I went to clozapine and that helped. You have to take the time to see which one works. It doesn't feel right in the beginning, but you have to find one that works. Clozapine works for me.

GENEVIVE: I hate pills because the medication is an illness of its own with the side effects. That's what I think about the medication. I've seen people with tardive dyskinesia, people with stiff limbs. It's another thing you have to deal with. You have to take the medication to feel better. You have no choice. Without it you'll have the symptoms. So you have to deal with the illness and with the medication. I have side effects: my menstruation does not come regularly, I'm lactating, I feel dizzy, and I can't stay up as late as I want. That's what I hate about it.

I don't like it one bit, but I need to stay on my feet. I need to go on with my life to accomplish my goal. In order for me to do that I have to take my medication or else I run the risk of relapsing, of getting sick again. And I don't want that because it's a setback.

RICHIE: The side effects I got were weight gain, drooling, feeling sluggish, stiffness. But it's like taking asthma medicine. If you have a disease with your lungs you have to take it. It's the same.

MEDICATION FOR THE REST OF MY LIFE?

Since everyone is different, you need to discuss with your doctor how long you will have to continue medication. The research done on the first episode of schizophenia shows that there is a high rate of relapse, which is usually related to discontinuing medication. The rate is five times higher in people who stop taking their medication.

This makes sense when you recall that schizophrenia is a chronic illness. That means—like diabetes or high blood pressure—it needs ongoing treatment to prevent symptoms from returning.

LUCINDA: I was about twenty-four when I got sick the first time. I always felt I was a very quiet person, quiet and normal, but very wary of people. I always found it very hard to trust people. I felt that people didn't like me, that people were against me except for close friends and my family. I don't want to think about the first time I got sick. It was a horrible experience. I felt very light. I felt like I was floating on air, like I wasn't part of the world. I just felt like I was floating. That was really the main feeling I had at the time, and it was scary.

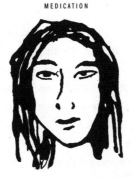

LUCINDA

My mother was diagnosed with manic depression. She had eleven children. She was hospitalized many times in her life, maybe every two years. But she found a good medication and she has been well—she hasn't been hospitalized the past eight years. I have never looked at my mother as "different."

When you are in the hospital with a mental illness, you don't feel good about it. You hope that things will get better when you get out, but having to take pills confirms, "Yes, you have a mental illness." This can be difficult. Taking pills is a reminder every day that "Yes, I am a sick person." Depending on the side effects of the medication, it can change your lifestyle. It can change what type of work you can do, and if people know you have this disease it can change the way they look at you. The sleepiness can change the job you have, or you may not be able to work as many hours as you had been. This can change your standard of living. I was fired from a couple of jobs because I wasn't on time.

I don't mind having to take medication for the rest of my life if I don't have the side effects. It's the side effects that are my main concern. I don't mind because there is always a chance of a cure for the illness, and then I won't have to take it.

MARCUS: I don't really like taking medication, but it helps me. I don't want to be on it forever. I want to get it reduced.

LINDA: The doctor said, "Well, in some instances people could come off in a year, but in most cases they stay on the medication." I felt good before I got sick, so I thought I was going to be one of those rare people. When I did get off the medication, I lost the weight that I gained and I had another nervous breakdown. They never told me it was for life.

AMBER: I feel that I don't want to take medication for the rest of my life. I hope that after a few years of not having symptoms I will talk with my doctor, and if I don't have any symptoms she will tell me I don't have to worry about taking medication. Right now it's like a habit, like popping a vitamin in the morning. Right now there is no hassle. I take it after dinner.

90

I don't think anybody wants to be on medication forever. I think I would like to have children one day. It might damage my chances of having a healthy baby. I don't know if that is true. Also, it would be great if I didn't have to remember to take medication all the time. It would be one less thing to think about.

VAN: It's not easy to remember to take the medication. It can make you feel like a patient. Ashamed. But the effects can be positive and can keep you out of the hospital.

I experienced drooling, sedation, and constipation. Besides getting the blood taken every week, I informed my doctor of my side effects and tried to do the best I could and realized that the medicine was doing its job. Mostly I was thankful that it was working, and I kind of accepted the side effects. I used to get so sedated I actually fell in the hospital a few times. I would not walk down stairs or drive.

MARK: Complaining about medication is good. I think the stupid thing is not taking it. You should ask your doctor. I don't like to be punished. I'm a very stubborn person. What the doctor did, he just gave me the percentages of relapse. If you look at that, your decisions are more emotion free, based on logic and common sense. You don't want to admit that you have a mental illness. Listen to your doctor's statistics—not his advice that your life is no different than it was before.

BEN: Taking medication becomes just part of your daily routine. I don't think about it. The way I figure it is that if the side effects hurt me in a really negative way, then I'll deal with it. I'm taking medicine now that totally doesn't affect me. I'm lucky now. All I have is a little tremor.

BETH: While I was upstate I stopped taking my medicine. Then I went to Texas and I was taking my medicine maybe one to three times a week. The last day I got full-blown paranoia, the full bit, and I wound up having to come home. Now I realize that I have to take it for the rest of my life. I would rather do that than deal with the consequences.

AUDREY: Someday I wish to be off the medication, but in a safe way. Sometimes I wonder how it is affecting me physically and what my life would be like without it. Sometimes I feel that it's somewhat unnatural to be changing the chemical makeup of my brain.

LAURIE: I like taking my pills. They make me better. I don't get upset about the weight. I just don't want to increase my medication or change it. I don't want to be sick. I don't want to have problems.

SAMANTHA: Unfortunately, the sad truth is that I'm going to have to be on medication for the rest of my life because I really do have the symptoms that I am taking the medication for.

BEAUX: Don't like it. Just sometimes I worry about side effects even though I've been lucky. You wonder if you are going to be on pills for the rest of your life. I guess if it doesn't do any physical harm to me it's okay. My goal is to try to be off in a couple of years. It's like a strategy. You want to move on; at the same time you don't get cocky that it won't happen again. You just hope it won't happen again. If I can't get off, I want to get down to the base minimum. I can accept that.

ALEXANDRA: Medication is awful because you have to take it all the time. It tastes awful. It's a hassle to remember when to take it and not take it. I'm gaining weight from it.

It's frightening because someday I would like to get married and I don't know if I can have children. If I don't have children in my life I will get very upset. I think the medications are bad for the baby.

THOMAS: Taking medication reminds me I am ill. Sometimes it bothers me because I don't feel like I am really sick. It just bothers me to take medicine.

VANESSA: I love pills. I don't think I would do without the medication. I take them every day. I don't miss a day. I was wondering if I will have to take medication for the rest of my life. If I have to I'll just do it, because I don't want to get sick again. I have two children, and I don't want them to see me in the hospital again.

SMOKEY: It sucks to have to take pills for the rest of my life. It makes you drowsy; you want to sleep.

MIKE: I didn't want to hear about taking medicine for the rest of my life—the fact that this illness is long term, that you don't know what to expect. It's kind of scary because you don't want it to come back. The fact that you have to take this medication for a long time means that it can come back.

It doesn't really bother me now. As long as I just keep taking the medicine and I don't get sick again. That's the main thing.

JACKIE: For the first couple of years taking medication, I hated the idea that I needed this pill to keep me stable. I hated that, so there were a few times that I stopped the medication on my own and got sick again. I hated the weight gain from the medication—that was another reason for stopping without the doctor's consent. I finally learned a little bit about medications, and my doctor allowed me to go on one that's weight neutral. I haven't lost any weight. But I really have just come to terms with it and accepted that I need it for the rest of my life. Now if I miss it I get nervous. I'll go out of my way to go home to take it because the last thing I want is to get sick again.

PATRICK: When I first started taking the medication I was a little discouraged because I thought I could get by with the least amount. But I watched some other people's side effects and thought, "I'm not so bad off"—drooling and drowsiness. Twenty minutes after I take it I fall right to sleep. It's good to take it right before bedtime. My appetite increased and I gained sixty or seventy pounds.

I wish someday I would be able to get off it. Be able to go back to my old self, trim. I wish I could get off it.

SHARON: Even in my younger years I didn't like taking pills, but thinking about having to take pills for the rest of my life—just the taste of them, the nasty aftereffect in your mouth. It tastes disgusting. Sometimes they are too big to swallow.

JAMES: I know I have to take it, so I take it. I get sick of swallowing those pills every day, but it's something you have to do. Just knowing that it's going to keep me healthy is the reason I like taking those pills. I've had weight gain, drooling on my pillow, constipation. At the beginning I couldn't wake up or it was hard to wake up, and I had to go to work. My reflexes at the beginning weren't like they were. And I used to get a lot of headaches, but taking the medicine took that away too.

It makes me feel better knowing the reason I take the medicine is that I won't be right otherwise. I don't really think about it. It's helping me out. It's like a habit, just taking it once a day. The blood work, though, is a pain in the neck.

LUCINDA: I stopped the medication because I was fired from my job. I was very tired and I wasn't getting up early in the morning to get to work. Work is very important to me. So I felt work came before medication, that it was better for me than medication. I believed I would be able to work without it. Not being able to hold a job was as much a fright as having a mental illness. I felt I wouldn't have been able to go on if I wasn't able to work. It was like a double blow. I decided to stop my medication. A lot changed in my life. My best friend went back to Scotland just then. I just started feeling very depressed, and I ended up back in the hospital. When I went home, I stopped it again. I was suicidal. I took overdoses.

ALEXIS: I love pills. I can lead a normal, functioning life. I went to college. I got a teaching job. I have forty children all day and eighty parents. I am getting my master's degree. I'm getting married. I'm able to maintain relationships with people. Without the medicine, I wasn't able to go to class. I would skip classes because I wasn't able to concentrate. I was not able to hold a relationship. I spent a lot of money that I didn't have. The doctor said I was unpleasant, not myself. I would talk so much I wouldn't let anybody get a word in, and people don't like that. Anybody who told me something I didn't want to hear, I wouldn't listen.

Complementary and Alternative Treatments

People sometimes look to other remedies for schizophrenia. Talk therapy, vitamins, and special diets are the major approaches people have tried—without much success.

TALK THERAPY Not so long ago people believed that "talk therapy" could cure schizophrenia. That made some sense when we believed schizophrenia was caused by the family environment. Now that we know that what causes schizophrenia is a biological problem, it is clear that we must help the brain recover with medicine. Although talking helps people cope with symptoms of schizophrenia, many well-done research studies tell us that talking does not take the place of medicine.

VITAMIN THERAPY Can vitamins take the place of medications? Some people, and even some doctors, think vitamins may be used to treat schizophrenia. Up until this writing there is no evidence to show that vitamins can replace antipsychotic medications for stopping hallucinations and delusions. But vitamins and minerals may be helpful for your overall health and possibly for mental functioning in general.

OMEGA-3 Fish-oil supplements containing omega-3 fatty acids (DHA and EPA acids) may have some real benefits in increasing focused thinking and in reducing depression. Omega-3 also may assist in reducing memory loss. Although research in these areas is not complete, there is reason to believe that taking fish-oil supplements, especially those with large amounts of EPA acid, can have positive effects on overall mental health. The direct benefit for symptoms of schizophrenia is not clear at this time, but it might help. The important thing to remember is to stay within recommended doses. Check with your doctor. Just because fatty acids and vitamins are sold without prescriptions does not mean they are always safe to take. In fact, fatty acids and vitamins are not regulated, so the best thing to do is to ask your doctor if fish oil is a good idea for you and, of course, how much to take. It is a good idea to show your doctor the bottle of fish oil so that he or she can check on the ingredients and advise you about the safest dose for you.

ANTIOXIDANTS A diet high in antioxidants is also thought to be good for everyone. Most fruits and vegetables contain antioxidants; berries and spinach have especially high amounts. Also, there are supplements that are good sources of antioxidants, such as Vitamin E and Vitamin C.

Remember, vitamins and other supplements sold without a prescription are not a cure for schizophrenia. Taking too much of a vitamin can be dangerous to your health. Get your doctor's advice before beginning vitamins and other supplements.

SPECIAL DIETS A healthy diet is essential for the optimal functioning of your whole body, including your brain. Diet fads are always around and this is no different for people with schizophrenia.

One new diet people are trying is the diet for people with celiac disease. Celiac disease is a disease of the digestive system. People who have it cannot tolerate the intake of gluten, a protein mostly found in wheat but also in barley and rye. The celiac diet does not cure schizophrenia or eliminate hallucinations and delusions. Still, some people believe there is a connection between celiac disease and schizophrenia and have tried this. The celiac diet is difficult to follow because it means eliminating all wheat products from your diet. Since there is no solid scientific evidence to show a connection between schizophrenia and celiac disease, it is best to speak to your doctor before you begin the celiac diet.

ELECTROCONVULSIVE THERAPY (ECT) Electroconvulsive therapy (ECT) has a long history. Many people think it is absolutely inhuman because of things they heard about it or saw in movies. Actually today it is very different: it is considered a very safe treatment for severe mood symptoms.

Sometimes, when medicine is not working effectively for psychotic symptoms, doctors recommend ECT. ECT causes changes to the chemistry of the brain that can help with many symptoms. Some people say it is like pressing a reset button in the brain.

What actually happens when you have ECT?

ECT today is different from the old days. First you are given anesthesia so that you sleep through the treatment. You will be given oxygen during the procedure. Electrodes that conduct electricity are placed on the head. A very small amount of electric current is applied to the brain for about thirty seconds so that you have a small, short seizure. For many people the seizure is so minor that all that happens is the big toe moves. That's it. The anesthesia is stopped, oxygen is removed and you go back to your room or home. Usually people sleep for a while afterward.

How many ECT treatments will I have?

How many treatments you will need varies. Usually it takes at least six treatments to see any changes. Your doctor will be the best judge of when to stop. If ECT helps you, your doctor may suggest you continue to have "booster" ECT, possibly once a month, to maintain the good effects of the treatment.

What are the side effects of ECT?

People often have some memory loss, especially memories around the time of the treatment. This is not fun but it is usually temporary. Some people do complain of memory loss for events going back several months. While this is not common, it does happen. Some people also complain about problems with their thinking, especially confusion. Again, for most people this disappears over time. Other possible immediate side effects are nausea, headache, and muscle ache—all of which are short-term problems your treatment team can help with.

Discuss ECT with your doctor to get more details.

For additional information about medications:

Medline Plus: www.nlm.nih.gov/medlineplus/

Check pharmaceutical company Web sites for detailed information regarding medications, side effects, and prescription assistance programs.

SafeMedication.com: www.safemedication.com/

NIMH: www.nimh.nih.gov/health/publications/mental-health-medications/ complete-index.shtml

Schizophrenia.com: www.schizophrenia.com provides a link to complementary treatments. Go to the main Web site and click on "schizophrenia treatment." From there click on "complementary therapies." This link will bring you to information about studies of complementary treatments. BEWARE: No one has yet proven that any of the complementary medications are beneficial. Speak to your treatment team and be very careful when considering complementary medication.

Partnership for Prescription Assistance: www.pparx.org/

OUT OF THE HOSPITAL AND STAYING WELL

At first it may seem that nothing could be harder than the hospital experience, but in the hospital there are many people helping you to recover. It's when you go home that you face the real challenge. You have more control over your life, which is good. But you also have many important decisions to make that will play a major role in your recovery.

You may have several options for follow-up treatment. It is not unusual to have some symptoms when you leave the hospital; if you do, you may need to attend a special program during the day. There are day programs and intensive outpatient programs that give you specialized treatment but allow you to sleep at home. Or you may be offered outpatient appointments with your psychiatrist and therapist.

When you make the choice to take advantage of follow-up treatment, you begin traveling down the road toward recovery. That road may have some bumps and curves. You will need to develop some good navigational skills to continue to stay on a healthy track and avoid relapse.

LINDA: I was twenty-three when it hit me. I was in college working on my degree, working part-time for the board of education. I had an obsessive, jealous boyfriend. It took me four years to break up with him. During those four years I wasn't allowed to talk to anyone. He always kept me like a caged bird. I felt trapped within myself. I had nowhere to go. He was my only key for survival. It was very difficult to be alone, a young girl alone

Special contributors: Julia Becker, M.D. and Steve Anderson, M.A.

trying to make something of herself. He stalked me the day I went to get an order of protection from him. He really scared me because he was always stalking me. I started having gynecological problems, so I called my gynecologist. His secretary said there were no appointments. After I hung up, something in my brain clicked. Her voice triggered something.

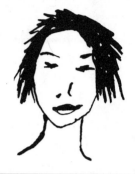

LINDA

I knew something was going on. I felt alive again for the first time in four years. I left work. I was in my apartment and started writing. I couldn't stop writing. Then my best friend called me up out of the blue. She was just great. I called my social worker from when I was a foster child. I was crying and crying. Then my mind started to race. I thought my boyfriend was sleeping with my roommate. I thought my roommate was killing my cats.

My parents had passed away. I couldn't go to my sister or my brother, so my last hope was the Blacks, my foster family. I hadn't talked to them in four years. I went back to them and they took me in. They cooked me dinner but I didn't eat it. I was 101 pounds, a twig. I hadn't eaten, slept, or gone to the bathroom in five days. All I could think of was that everyone was out to get me. I thought my friends were talking about me. The only people I trusted were my brother, my sister, and the Blacks. I was having these hallucinations, seeing people who weren't there. The main man I was focusing on was my art professor. It had been love at first sight. But he was my professor and I was a student. I started calling him up and harassing him. When he didn't respond, I thought he was "in on it." My sister told me to stop calling him. I was leaving him notes under his office door. I even followed him one time. Then he threw me out of his class and told me he was going to call security. There was this guy in the class I liked. I was trying to get his number from information in the middle of the night. In my effort to get the number from information I was screaming. Mrs. Black woke up and called 911. The police took me to the hospital. When they locked me in a room, I started kicking the door. It took five men to keep me down. They gave me a shot, and I fell asleep. The next thing I knew, I was in a gown in a wheelchair. It's scary. I stayed in the hospital for fourteen days. When I went home I took myself off the medication. My symptoms were coming back. I did a lot of crying and I was very angry.

99

I now know what happened to me. It took me five years to accept it and adjust to my medications. I used to cry. I wouldn't even mind surgery. I wish I could have had anything rather than a mental illness, but now I am accepting it.

ACCEPTANCE

Acceptance of your illness will come slowly but not steadily. One day you accept and the next you deny. This is a normal response to any serious illness. Talk about your feelings regarding your diagnosis. Talk to your group members, your therapist, your doctor, your family, and close friends. Don't let a relapse force you to get help.

BETH: I didn't believe it was going to be for the rest of my life. I was hoping that it was going to be the schizophreniform diagnosis and it wasn't going to continue. So I wound up stopping my medicine. It would make me tired, and I didn't want to take it because I didn't think I would have to.

BEN: With this illness, reaching the point of self-awareness is very important. That means acknowledging that you are sick. If other people try to help, you have to let them. Accepting that you have the illness is very important. If you think, "I only have to take the drugs till I feel better," it doesn't work. Accept the truth and move on.

BUDDY: It has a lot to do with the individual being willing to get help. If the individual is not willing, then the family has to be involved.

JACKIE: A few times I felt sorry for myself and just cried, but I didn't like feeling that way. I realized I could have a normal life even though I went through this, even if I have to stay on medication. I don't regret anything from the past. I'm almost glad my life went the way it did. I'm happy with my life now.

LUCINDA: Realize it's not a life-threatening illness, like cancer or heart disease, and you can lead a good life on your medication. Talk with people who understand your illness, like those people that have the same illness as you, and your doctors and social workers.

One Day at a Time

Sometimes it seems like you will never be where you want to be. It feels like getting well takes forever. At those times, recall other times when you thought you would never get to your goal, like graduating from elementary school or getting over the flu. It does take a long time to heal, but remember, it will get better. Meanwhile, take one day at a time.

ILAN: I know it's a cliché, but take it one day at a time. What I learned from my counselor is that many of us can't see a light at the end of the tunnel. I always saw a light, and the light helped me. I didn't always know that I would reach it, but having it out there kept me going. It didn't clear away every problem. I also knew that every time you get punched down you have to get up. Parts of my immediate family were very supportive. I had them to hold me up at times. I had a good social network, people I could continually count on. Also, if you lose a friend, whether it is over your illness or not, you are bound to find another one as long as you are open to it.

And don't forget to breathe. Sometimes I cry and sometimes I take a deep breath, and sometimes I stare directly into space, better known as the television. I cried this morning. I don't think it makes me weak. It's a kind of therapy. Then I get up and I breathe. Music helps; it's a bit of an escape.

One Step at a Time

When the severe symptoms begin to disappear, it is time to get back into your life. At first you will not be quite ready to go to school or work. After all, if you were recovering from any other serious illness you would not go right back to your old schedule. You would be encouraged to start gradually, one step at a time.

LINDA: Get up, force yourself into the shower. Do not go back to bed after that alarm rings. Then get into that shower. Try to exercise and eat a healthy diet. Exercise your mind. Read the newspaper in the morning. Read a book at night. Watch a movie. Meditate. Listen to the radio. Play with your dog or get a cat. Talk to a friend. Go to school, to a program, to work. Have a structured routine. Every morning, get up at the same time. Get enough sleep, at least seven or eight hours a night.

SAMANTHA: I try to keep myself as busy as possible, occupied with things and activities that I enjoy. I try to focus my attention on other people at times.

GENEVIVE: Take the meds and then set a goal for yourself, something you are going to work toward.

ILAN: Just go on with your life. Because at the beginning you think you are some crazy person, and your self-esteem can get low. I think seeing a social worker helps me. I like exercising and feeling good. So do whatever it takes to help you keep your self-esteem up. So, what helps you to keep your self-esteem high?

BEN: It's part of life. You make the best of what you have. Play with the cards you are dealt. You can make things like this work for you. A lot of people, when they are at a disadvantage, they excel.

STAYING CONNECTED TO TREATMENT

Treatment means going to your doctor, who will monitor your medication. It also means going to a day program or to therapy. Some people go to group psychotherapy while others attend individual sessions. Having a group or a therapist with whom you can discuss anything at all about your illness and your goals is a big step toward staying well.

ALEXIS: When I was eighteen, I knew something was wrong. It started before I even got sick. I shoplifted and I got arrested. About two months after that, I got so scared I was going to go to jail that I didn't feel right. I lost my concentration when I was reading my schoolwork, and I noticed that my arm was hurting. I called the social worker at the time and I went in for a visit. He said it was just a panic attack, but I wanted to go to the hospital. So my mom and I went over to the hospital and I stayed overnight. The next day they took me from Coney Island Hospital to Kings County Hospital. I was scared of the "big nurse." I was there for five weeks, and I thought I was going to die. I kept saying, "Am I dying, am I dying?" I hallucinated that I was raped. I felt very stiff from the medicine, so stiff that I couldn't move at one point. The hospital was very depressing during the day, and we would just sit. That made the days seem very long. The only activity you could do was pace up and down the hallway. Then I was transferred to Hillside. I didn't want to take a shower for weeks. I just didn't want to get out of bed. My feet kept moving—like a march. I couldn't read because I couldn't concentrate, and my arms were so stiff I thought I would never drive again. Most of the time I couldn't sleep at night. When I was in the hospital I thought that I was there because I stole. I didn't understand then that the stealing was just a losing-your-judgment type of thing. I did feel scared, and I thought I would never get better. I told my mother to sell the car. I just thought I was dying.

You have to want to get well. I have to take the medicine to stay well. I wouldn't be where I am today without the medicine. I tried, and I can't go off it. The therapist and doctor are there to help me, but I have to come to help myself. Therapy is a two-way street.

ILAN: I think that therapy gave me a great deal of self-esteem and self-confidence. It also made me feel comfortable with myself. Within therapy there are boundaries. It also helps you understand other people better as well as yourself. You can make small but very important decisions based on things you learn in therapy. You are better as a person, healthier mentally when you can understand other people. My friends come to me sometimes now because they know I will hear them out and I'll listen to all sides of the story. Group therapy helps other people too, because you are giving support to others from what you've learned. It's a good boost, and it also helps the stress level.

JAMES: The groups help a lot because I'm talking with a lot of other people who have the same problems. Just the fact that you are going to the meetings is keeping you busy. And the doctors and the therapist you have are there to help. Coming to the hospital, it's like the only place you can really get down and talk about it because you are with people who went through the same thing. Every time I left a meeting I felt good; I was in a good mood. The times that I wouldn't go or didn't feel like going, those were the times I wouldn't feel too good. Once I got to the meeting I could talk about everything.

ROMAN: Go to group therapy. Stay on your medication.

ALEXANDRA: Now I come to Hillside every week. I come to see my therapist, nurse, and doctor. I see the nurse about the clozapine medicine. I see Dr. Becker for my other two medicines. I come to see Mrs. Miller for more counseling and to talk about what I've been doing and setting goals. Tomorrow I'm going to an interview at Citiview Connections. I hope they can try to get me a volunteer or part-time job, whichever comes first. I want to learn more about computers, learn how to get there, and make new friends.

Day Programs

Day programs are very helpful to many people who do not need treatment in the hospital unit but still need some extra help. Many day programs will help you with plans for school or work when you are ready.

LAURIE: Being in the day program is like you have a lot of friends and teachers who are really nice. They are always there to be a friend to you. I like the classes; you get to cook and talk about anything you want. It helps having something to do every day until I get well. They helped me with getting into college.

BEN: Everyone is different. The day hospital works, although people keep denying, saying, "I don't want to go." I was one of them. A lot of times when doctors, social workers, or counselors tell you something, you just have to stick with it because at the time you don't realize it's beneficial for you. Later when you look back you will thank God that they were very persistent. But that's the thing—a lot of times, so many factors have to work together.

BUCK: I would say take your medication. Listen to your therapists. If you are in a program, do the activities they have for you in the rehabilitation process.

DECREASING STRESS

Doctors do not believe that stress causes schizophrenia, but once you have schizophrenia, stress can affect your health. This is true of many other illnesses. For example, people with diabetes or heart disease are more likely to develop some symptoms when under too much stress.

When you work to keep your stress level at a minimum, you are helping to keep the chemistry of the brain from becoming imbalanced.

MEREDITH: I try to stay away from stressful things that will make it worse. Every time I think I'm going to be sick, I get more selfish for myself instead of taking care of other people.

I think more about what I want than what everyone else wants. I think more about who I am and what I need to do to stay healthy. I'm more aware of other people's pain. I'm learning now to avoid negative people and negative situations and learning how to deal with them. And after everything I've been through, I can still have hope for my future.

GARY: I talk more about other things that are giving me stress, am a little bit more talkative with my family and my friends, see my therapist and psychiatrist.

ALEXIS: Don't take on too much stress at one time. It might take a little longer to do something, but you will get it done. It's good to build up gradually. If you get overwhelmed, nothing will get done. Do deep breathing exercises.

AMBER: Be around people you like to be around. I spend a lot of time with my family. We like to eat out, Indian food, Korean food. I do a lot of things with my friends. We go shopping, have lunch, or just hang out at my friend's house.

> Because schizophrenia is an illness, it is important that you *sleep well, eat well,* and *exercise regularly.* Likewise, it is important that you *socialize, date,* and *visit with family* as soon as you can tolerate it. Ask your treatment team to help you plan this. —Julia Becker, M.D.

DATING

Dating and intimate relationships are an important part of life. It may take time to begin relationships again, but this is part of returning to healthy living. It is best to meet people through friends and family, in school, or at work. There are many Web sites for dating. However, like everyone else, you will need to be extremely careful using the Web to meet people. Sometimes it is easier to date someone who also has a mental illness. You may want to ask your therapist or NAMI for help locating dating services that specialize in people with mental illnesses.

VAN: I think initially it's challenging to kind of get back into the dating scene, but you should realize that it could help in your recovery because it can make you realize that you have recovered and that you still have the need to be with someone. I think it is important to date. I also think that your treatment and your diagnosis shouldn't be the topic of conversation on the date. At first it was difficult to get myself over thinking that I was in this place, that I was sick, and that I was on medication. When I put that aside and I was myself and would talk to someone, I would enjoy seeing who I was again and enjoy it. That made me feel a lot better. I think that's a big step in recovery.

BETH: Dating is normal, the same as for anybody else. It's difficult when you get sick, though. My relationship with my first boyfriend ended after I became ill. We didn't even stay friends. My new boyfriend knew about it beforehand. It's in his family too. He was very understanding and it didn't matter to him.

RELAPSE

A relapse occurs when symptoms that were once completely gone or under control begin to appear again. Sometimes people experience brief episodes of symptoms that come and then quickly disappear. We call these "blips." Many relapses can be stopped with help from your treatment team. The sooner you let your doctor know about symptoms, the better.

AMBER: When you have symptoms, tell your doctor. Maybe she can raise your medication so the symptoms don't recur. For example, the minute you notice that you are seeing things or hearing things that aren't there, tell your doctor.

GENEVIVE: I just don't let symptoms bother me as much because I know it's an illness. I try hard not to think about them. Now when I'm sad I know it's my illness. I know I don't have to do something drastic. I can try to do something to come out of it. I do the breathing exercises. I watch TV, play music. I kind of lift myself up from the depression that I'm getting. When they lowered my meds and I started to get symptoms, I made sure my doctor knew about it. I had my olanzapine dose raised. I was doing a lot better with it. When I'm feeling sad, I tell my father or my mother or my sister. They always tell me I have nothing to feel sad about. I think maybe they don't understand that when I'm sad it is part of my illness.

MEREDITH: Relapse is very frustrating because you depend on the medication to work. It works most of the time, but there's a chance you'll just get sick. It's not anyone's fault. You have this illness. It may not work the way you want. You just have to live with the highs and lows. It doesn't mean it's always going to be there. But it makes you aware of the precious moments, how wonderful the little things, how great the big things. And you just keep moving on.

106

> *Know the Signs of Relapse*
>
> It is helpful to know your own warning signs so that you can get help as early as possible. Some early warning signs may be changes in appetite, weight loss, decreased or increased sleep, disturbed sleep, or changes in energy level. There may also be symptoms such as paranoia, feeling people are looking at you, or a return of other symptoms you experienced previously. As soon as you notice a change or a new symptom, it is very important to call your doctor. The doctor may be able to adjust the medication to prevent further symptoms and avoid hospitalization. If it is too uncomfortable to speak with the doctor, talk to a family member or therapist to get help. — Julia Becker, M.D.

ILAN: While I was in day hospital the first time, the doctors were telling me they believed my diagnosis wasn't exactly schizophrenia. It was "brief reactive psychosis," and that meant that it was a schizophrenialike breakdown where I had the illness and it was gone. They believed this because I was able to get better from the medication so quickly. I remember, I think it was the last day of day hospital, my father came to pick me up. I said, "I'm free," and I really thought this was the end because they took me off the medication. I really wanted to believe it.

After some time passed, manic symptoms began to surface that nobody noticed, including me. I was buying a lot of things I didn't need. I had no space for this stuff. My bedroom looked like someone had pushed all of the things from the rest of my apartment into one room. My thoughts on the matter were that I bought furniture to start my own apartment. The only problem was, it was enough furniture for a two-bedroom apartment.

As for the second breakdown, I remember I was in class in college and was kicked out of two classes. This breakdown was different. I was in the emergency room and I wasn't screaming or anything. They were able to bring me in without strapping me down. But I was delusional. At the hospital they interviewed me, and I noticed the pause in the writer's hands as she was trying to make sense of what I said so she could chart it. After more breakdownlike behavior, I was admitted to Low III. It becomes a little vague. I was in the quiet room. I still didn't know what was going on because I thought I was there to help other people. When I was finally discharged, I really didn't want to go back to day hospital because it was a living hell. But I realized I wasn't going to win. I went through day hospital and started vocational rehab. At that point my doctor took me off the Prolixin, after I had only been put back on for five months.

The next break came when I was at synagogue. It was my holiday, Passover, and I was praying with the congregation. I realized for the first time that my thoughts were going quickly. I couldn't concentrate on one thought alone. They were jumping from one to another. I made it through the holiday and the festive meals because I thought it was important to do so. My father returned from my stepmom's family and I told him in a way that I thought would be easy on him, let him know I was getting sick again. Finally I said, "Dad, I'm going down. I need to go to the hospital tomorrow." That was the last hospitalization—four years ago.

AUDREY: The first thing is to be completely honest with your doctors about your symptoms. Also, being aware of your symptoms in order to prevent relapse is very important.

JEFF: Early signs: not sleeping, worrying about stuff that didn't happen.

ALEXIS: Recognize your symptoms—mine are talking too much, spending too much, not sleeping, not eating. And then get help.

BETH: Every time that I've gotten sick, I've had anxiety before.

Tips on Preventing Relapse

Staying well can be more difficult than getting well. Most times this is because of problems with the medication or skipping doses, but sometimes it is due to mistakes in taking care of the stressors that can interfere with recovery. Sticking with the treatment, abstaining from drugs and alcohol, having structure, getting good sleep, and making time for enjoyment are all important elements in staying well.

ZELDA: To stay well, you never give in to actions that you know may cause harm. For instance, I know that I can't stay up really late. So one night I'll stay up till four o'clock, but the rest of the month I know I have to stay on track. So give yourself a little slack, but not too much.

LINDA: Go to therapy. Talk to a friend. Go to school, to a program, to work. Have a structured routine. Every morning, get up at the same time. Get enough sleep, at least seven or eight hours a night. Of course you are going to take your medicine, that's a given. And take it at the same time each day.

VANESSA: I take my medication every day. And if I run out I call the doctor. I try to eat right. I try to get out with my friends now. The doctors in the hospital helped me. My mother and my father, especially my mother, helped me. I know I have to take care of myself. I know I have to see the doctor on a regular basis. My therapy also, I have to have that. That helps a lot.

LUCINDA: To stay well, my advice would be to continue taking the medication. Stay away from people who like to upset you. Keep yourself busy so you have less time to think about your illness. Don't think about having a mental illness, just carry on with life. Work if at all possible, even part time, because you'll feel more like a normal person if you are working.

JACKIE: Over the past few years I've been experimenting with what to do to keep myself well. I stopped drinking alcohol and I've stayed well ever since. I try to keep a structured life with a schedule so I have things to do. That keeps me focused rather than in a dreamy world.

Helpful Medication Tips

INVEST IN A MEDICATION REMINDER BOX The see-through boxes are the best. Fill it once a week to help you keep track. When you fill it and see you will run out soon, get a refill immediately.

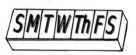

KEEP TRACK OF YOUR MEDICATION HISTORY Use the medication log at the end of this chapter or get a notebook to enter each time you get a new medication. If possible, also keep track of dose changes.

If your doctor changes your medication, write down the reason. That way you may prevent unnecessarily retrying a medication that causes you problems or does not work.

Healthy Habits

VAN: Keeping busy, continuing with medication, continuing with therapy, continuing communication, family support, decreasing things that make you anxious, using breathing exercises—that's one of the best things.

SAMANTHA: I attend my groups, I talk to my counselors, I talk to my parents, and I take my medication. I do what I need to do for myself. I always ask my mom, "How do you see my behavior? Is anything amiss?" Medication helps me stay well; seeing my doctor and therapist regularly; checking in with the apartment program as needed.

BEN: You need a routine. Medicine. You can't be erratic about sleep and exercise. If you do a little research you learn that not sleeping is the first symptom for a lot of people. I constantly seek to improve myself, and in doing that I learn more about myself and how to be a better person. When you know yourself you have some control. This means also to know yourself physically, how you are feeling. You are more aware, and that's really important.

Here is a list of our "top thirteen" tips to staying well:

Take mediation as prescribed.

Go to your therapy sessions.

Keep your doctor appointments.

Reduce stress.

Take one step at a time.

Do enjoyable activities.

Do not use drugs or alcohol.

Get plenty of sleep with a regular sleep schedule.

Eat foods that are healthy.

Exercise ten to twenty minutes each day.

Talk with your family and friends.

Know your own warning signs.

Build a routine into your days.

TREATMENT AND REHABILITATION PROGRAMS

Medications are the foundation for recovery, but most people benefit from additional treatments, which are generally called psychosocial treatments. In fact, combining medication and psychosocial treatment is well known to get the best results. Psychosocial treatment is provided when you are in the hospital, in the day hospital, and out of the hospital as well. There are many types of psychosocial treatments, all of which are helpful in varying ways at different stages of recovery. And they are all aimed at helping you regain your health and independence.

110   *Case management* services help to coordinate treatment. You may be assigned a case manager who helps you get benefits, find a doctor or a treatment program, and tackle numerous other practical needs you may have as you recover. Since finding your way around the complex medical system can be extremely hard, your case manager may prove to be a key person in your treatment.

Cognitive behavioral treatment (CBT) can be used in many ways to address problems of thinking and behaviors related to your thoughts. CBT training helps to build new coping skills that can be used for numerous difficulties, such as keeping your mood steady, dealing with negative thoughts, improving your attention as you return to school or work, and decreasing use of substances.

Cognitive enhancement treatment (CET), *Cognitive remediation (CR)*, and *Cognitive adaptation training (CAT)* are treatment approaches designed to decrease difficulties with cognition, primarily attention, learning, memory, and problem solving. There are a variety of approaches to improving cognition, most of which involve practice and finding new ways to approach each individual's cognitive problems. There is a great deal of research now into finding the best ways to improve cognition. We know now that the brain is a lot like a muscle: the more you use it the stronger it gets.

Double-trouble groups are self-help groups for people with mental illness and substance abuse problems. These groups are run by the consumers with a goal of helping each other give up substances in order to maximize recovery from mental illness. These are special groups run in a similar way as Alcoholics Anonymous groups. Ask your treatment team for information on where to find a double-trouble group.

Family treatments come in several forms. There is psychoeducation for families, just as there is psychoeducation for you. Then there are family groups that may or may not include you. Many people like family groups where members from several families meet together. These are called multiple family groups. But sometimes you may meet with just your family and a therapist or case manager. In all cases, the goal of family treatment is to decrease the problems that you and your family may be experiencing.

Group or individual psychotherapy provides a supportive environment for working on issues of recovery. The therapist will not be exploring your past family issues but will be working with you or the group to move toward reaching your goals. This treatment may include segments on psychoeducation, skills training, CBT, and healthy lifestyles. Most important is that you feel supported and safe to discuss your concerns with your group or individual therapist.

Integrated treatment for people with schizophrenia recognizes that having a dual diagnosis of schizophrenia and substance abuse requires a very specialized approach. The therapist is fully aware that your medications are required to maintain your mental health and that you may experience significant stress as you give up substance use. The therapist will help you address both issues at the same time.

Psychoeducation helps you learn about your illness and its treatment. This is very important because if you do not understand schizophrenia, it may be difficult to make the healthiest decisions about your self-care. This book contains a great deal of psychoeducation, but it is always better to have someone to answer questions and support you as you learn about this very complicated illness called schizophrenia.

Self-help groups are very effective for some people and have been beneficial for people with substance abuse and other problems for many years. It is wonderful to be with peers who really understand your concerns. It is less costly, and best of all, you are doing it on your own. Finding self-help groups is getting easier on the Internet.

Social clubs, drop-in centers, clubhouses, and advocacy groups are wonderful places to find friends, enjoyable activities, and support. Your case manager will be able to guide you to the best social clubs and drop-in centers in your area. NAMI has information on its Web site regarding its Peer-to-Peer program. NAMI is also a powerful advocate for the rights of people with mental illnesses. See the section on clubhouses for additional information.

Social skills training targets problems interacting with people that may develop due to schizophrenia. This training will help you rebuild your ability to communicate and build relationships with those around you. If you notice that you have difficulty keeping a conversation going, being assertive, meeting new people, or interviewing for school or jobs, social skills training could be just the thing for you.

Vocational rehabilitation is important for helping you return to school or work. See chapter 17 for a full description of vocational rehabilitation.

Additional resources:

Self-help program listings: www.mentalhelp.net/selfhelp/

NAMI: nami.org

Compeer: www.compeer.org/

National Mental Health Consumers' Self-Help Clearinghouse: www. mhselfhelp.org

Secret handshake support group: www.thesecrethandshake.ca/

Dealing with Cognitive Dysfunction Associated with Psychiatric Disabilities, by A. Medalia and N. Revheim, Office of Mental Health, New York State; www.omh.state.ny.us/omhweb/cogdys_manual/cogdyshndbk.htm.

Cognitive Enhancement Therapy for Schizophrenia. Effects of a Two-Year Randomized Trial on Cognition and Behavior, by Hogarty et al. *Archives of General Psychiatry*, 2004.

"Psychosocial Rehabilitation Services in Community Support Systems: A Review of the Outcomes and Policy Recommendations," by R. Barton, *Psychiatric Services* 50, no. 4 (1999); www.psychservices.psychiatryonline.org/cgi/content/full/50/4/525.

TREATMENT MODELS

Psychosocial treatment is provided in many different ways. Several popular models of treatment—the clubhouse model, assertive community treatment, and the recovery model—are just a few ways people have organized treatment to provide help.

Clubhouse Model

The clubhouse model was developed at Fountain House, a nonprofit organization in New York City, in the 1940s. Through a training program started at Fountain House in 1976, this model has now spread to more than 350 other such facilities around the world.

The clubhouse model, based on the conviction that mental illness is not the whole person and that people with mental illness retain the same needs, capabilities, and aspirations as all other people, is made up of a network of communities. Each community is situated in a clubhouse building where people who seek services participate as members. The community is organized to promote the recovery of members from schizophrenia, bipolar disorder, major depression, and other serious and persistent forms of mental illness.

Participation by members is voluntary. All clubhouse services are provided by the members and staff, who work side by side as colleagues. At the core of the clubhouse experience is the work-ordered day, which intentionally parallels the typical business hours of the general adult community. Together, members and staff prepare daily meals, operate the switchboard, issue a newsletter, run the mailroom, operate an employment placement and support program, manage housing and housing support services, participate in advocacy efforts on behalf of people with mental illness, and accomplish other projects to benefit the life of the clubhouse.

In addition, clubhouses provide support for members who wish to have access to opportunities available in the larger society. Clubhouse-operated transitional employment programs comprise agreements between clubhouses and employers through which members can obtain supported, competitive employment. Supported education programs in clubhouses enable members to return to college or other schools according to their interests, needs, and goals. Clubhouses assist members in acquiring decent housing; many operate housing programs.

The length of clubhouse membership extends for as long as each person wishes. In this way, ongoing support and opportunity, as well as case management and planning, are provided on a consistent and continuous basis. Clubhouses also operate evening and weekend programs, which focus on social and recreational activities and also allow members who are working full-time or are in school during the day to maintain involvement. Members who withdraw or are rehospitalized are encouraged to return through outreach contacts. In all cases, clubhouses focus on members' strengths, talents, and abilities, providing a place to explore and celebrate, as well as enabling members to rebuild careers and relationships that may have been disrupted by disabling illness.

To find a clubhouse model program in your area:

Call 1–212–582–0343

Write to International Center for Clubhouse Development at 425 W. 47 St., New York, New York 10036

Check the ICCD Web site at www.iccd.org.

Assertive Community Treatment Model (ACT)

Assertive community treatment is available in some areas of the United States, Canada, and Great Britain. What makes ACT unique is that if you are treated by an ACT team you have 24-hour service available right in your community. ACT teams offer case workers, psychiatric services, help with housing, family support, and many of the various other supports you may benefit from. Do not hesitate to take advantage of an ACT team if it is available to you.

Get more information about ACT from NAMI at www.nami.org or contact The ACT Association at 810–227–1859 or acta@actassociation.org.

Recovery Model

The recovery model is based on the idea that all people with schizophrenia and other illnesses that affect the mind deserve the opportunity to live as well as they can. This means that even when a person's symptoms have not fully gone away, he or she can go to work, go to school, have close relationships, and behave just about the same as before illness. In this way, the recovery model can be seen as promoting hopefulness and helping people feel confident and—overall—good about themselves as they are working to recover. It can also be thought of as a way of reducing prejudices from those who do not understand what it is like to have schizophrenia. The Recovery Model is also used for people with addictions to alcohol, marijuana, and drugs.

Important to know: All models of treatment, including the recovery model, stress a team approach between consumers and clinicians. This means that you and your psychiatrist work out a medication plan together. It is never a good idea to stop or change doses of medication without first discussing your plan with your doctor.

For more information on the recovery model, check out these Web sites and books:

www.surgeongeneral.gov/library/mentalhealth/chapter2/sec10.html

www.socialworkers.org/practice/behavioral_health/0206snapshot.asp

Recovery and Wellness, Models of Hope and Empowerment for People with Mental Illness, Mary Donohue and Catana Brown (Haworth Press, 2001).

The Healing Journey through Addiction, Phil Rich and Stuart Copans (Wiley, 2000).

INVOLUNTARY COMMITMENT

114

Sometimes people are treated for psychiatric illnesses against their will. Involuntary treatment may be in the form of inpatient hospitalization or outpatient doctor visits as ordered by the court. The laws vary greatly from state to state in the United States, but in general involuntary commitment only happens when it appears someone may be a danger to her/himself or to other people. Anyone who is involuntarily committed has the right to go to court. If the court believes you need to be committed (inpatient or outpatient), you will be required to follow the court's directions for treatment. If the court disagrees with your commitment, you will be free to make your own decisions about treatment.

Clearly no one wants to be forced to be in treatment. One way people take back some control is by use of psychiatric advance directives and by assigning a health care agent. People can make decisions about their care or have someone they trust to have their best interests in mind involved in treatment decisions during episodes of psychosis.

For additional information:

Check your state's Web site for involuntary commitment laws.

Office of Mental Health (OMH) for each state

Bazelon Center for Mental Health Law: www.bazelon.org

Mental Health America: www.nmha.org/go/position-statements/p-36

ADVANCE DIRECTIVES

Sometimes people do not have a lot of warning before a relapse. It is a good idea to ask your doctor about getting an advance directive, which is a written statement about what you do and don't want to happen if you become ill and are unable to make decisions. Advance directives in psychiatry allow doctors to make important treatment decisions when you are not well enough to do so on your own. If, for example, you get sick and your thoughts are confused or you are hearing voices, you may not be well enough to make important choices about taking medication, doses, or even whether you should be admitted to the hospital. At such times, advance directives can help.

There are two types of psychiatric advance directives. The first type is the instruction directive. When you are well, you write out clear instructions about your treatment to be followed at times when you cannot think clearly. Instruction directives are similar to living wills, in which people write out in advance their instructions about future medical treatment.

The second type is the proxy directive, *also known as the* medical power of attorney. This assigns someone you trust as a substitute decision maker for times when you are unable to make decisions for yourself. Often, people combine instruction directives and proxy directives into one document so they are assured the best possible care that they would want for themselves.

Advance psychiatric directives are accepted in some form in all fifty states, but certain states are more strongly committed to the concept than others. Also, because these directives are legally complicated, it is best to have a lawyer draw one up for you in the state where you live. You may be entitled to a free legal aid attorney in your community, or you may visit a law clinic; they are frequently found near universities that have law schools. The National Association of Protection and Advocacy Systems (NAPAS) can supply you with information about your state's laws by referring you to your local NAPAS office. You can call them at (202) 408–9514. There is also information available on the Web at www.napas.org. The National Alliance for the Mentally Ill (NAMI) frequently includes articles about advance directives on their legal Web site. An interesting, easy-to-read article can be found at www.nami.org/legal/advanced.html. Additional information and examples of legal forms can be found at www.bazelon.org/advdir.html. If you do not have access to the Internet, ask your case manager or clinician to help you access this information.

Additional resources:

The Complete Family Guide to Schizophrenia, by Kim Meuser and Susan Gingerich (Gillford, 2006), especially chapter 12 on making a relapse plan.

NIMH, "Recovery After an Initial Schizophrenia Episode (RAISE): A Research Project of the NIMH," www.nimh.nih.gov/health/topics/schizophrenia/raise/index.shtml

National Mental Health Consumers' Self-Help Clearinghouse: www.mhselfhelp.org

Me, Myself, and Them: A Firsthand Account of One Young Person's Experience with Schizophrenia, by Kurt Snyder, Raquel E. Gur, and Linda Wasmer Andrews (Oxford University Press, 2007).

FEMA, Americans with Disabilities Act of 1990 (ADA): www.fema.gov/oer/reference/ada_1990.shtm; 2008 version: www.ada.gov/pubs/ada.htm

MEDICATION LOG

Enter medication changes in your log along with side-effects and reasons for changing medications. (see page #.)

DATE	MEDICATION	SIDE-EFFECTS/REASON FOR DISCONTINUATION

117

MEDICATION LOG

DATE	MEDICATION	SIDE-EFFECTS/REASON FOR DISCONTINUATION

10

COPING WITH POSITIVE AND NEGATIVE SYMPTOMS

Each person's symptoms improve at different rates. Often the hallucinations and delusions decrease more quickly than other symptoms. You may have problems with simple things like getting out of bed, brushing your teeth, or connecting with other people. With treatment and hard work, the obstacles to getting back to your old self become less overwhelming.

The best way to get help with your symptoms is to consult your treatment team. They will know your individual needs. However, we have included some suggestions that helped us cope with the symptoms we experienced. For definitions of positive and negative symptoms, see chapter 4.

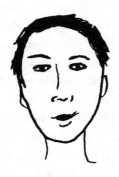

MIKE

MIKE: I am twenty years old. I knew that I had a sickness around June of last year. I was very hyper. I felt I had special powers and I felt I was in another world, a whole different world. I was seeing hallucinations, different types of animals, dragons, and all different types of things. It felt as if there were a plot, demons or evil out to get me. I was hearing voices and just basically worried that something was going to happen to my family. It felt like the government might have been in on it. Like the TV was talking to me. Any show that was on, it was talking to me. If I was watching cartoons, like if *Batman* was on, Batman and I were joining forces to destroy the evil that was out to get me. My emotions were very high. I was on a natural high, like nothing could take me down. I was unconquerable. I talked more. It was a very happy feeling. Then I felt real sick and I just got real close within myself.

I was at Adelphi University. I wanted to play volleyball, but there was a class in the gym. They asked me to leave, and I wouldn't leave. From that point on I just started getting withdrawn into myself. I wouldn't leave the court because I wanted to play my game and I felt people just didn't want to see me playing my game. After that I was put in handcuffs and taken down to the station. I felt this was all a setup, part of the plot against me. When I got to the station I just completely blocked out from everybody. It was like I wasn't even in my body. I was unconscious.

That night I ended up at the county hospital, and it was like I was being attacked inside my brain and nobody could help me. It was like I was being closed off from the natural world. So that night they gave me some type of tranquilizer to try to calm me down. I was out of it for a couple of hours and they didn't know what was wrong. After a while I woke up and I just wasn't calm. So they gave me another tranquilizer. I was on Ativan, and it helped to keep me calm. It gave me a good feeling.

A few days later I met Dr. Hoffman and Mrs. Miller and went for some visits talking to different doctors. They found out that I had a chemical imbalance. Then I went in for treatment at the hospital. I was tested, different kinds of tests, on computers, blood tests, people asking me questions. The doctors there and the social worker were treating me. I was in Low III for three or four weeks. While I was there it was pretty good. I didn't feel that I was myself at that time, but after a while things were getting clearer. I was taking medication. I was eating more, which I wasn't doing before.

After a while I was released and most of my symptoms were gone—seeing things, hearing voices—all those things were gone. But from going through the illness I had a depression, I was very sad. I went through this whole ordeal. I felt as though I wasn't prepared to go on with life. Like all my dreams were beaten out of me through this illness. Then I went into the aftercare program and the whole staff there helped me learn how to start over. And that's what you have to do, start over again with your relationships with other people, taking care of yourself hygienewise, making sure you look good, and building up your self-confidence again.

I was in the aftercare program starting over, and I was learning more about my illness, how to cope with it, how to deal with it, not to be in denial. I went to different group sessions. I had group therapy with the social worker. At first I didn't think that these groups would be able to help me. I didn't think I was getting anything out of them. But then I found out that there are other people who can relate to what I've been through, and I can relate to them too. So that helped me out a lot, being able to have something in common with other people there. Time went on. I got better. My depression level went down. I began to feel like myself, not totally, but almost there.

It's still pretty difficult. I try to make up different schedules. I try working out to get more energy during the day. I try to discipline myself to get up early, to get things going. I put little reminders up on the wall, things I have to do during the day, any little thing I have to do. I keep trying to let my family know what I want to accomplish so that they can help me out if they see that I'm not doing it.

COPING WITH POSITIVE SYMPTOMS OF PSYCHOSIS

The only effective way to deal with positive symptoms is to take your medication. But it can take time for the medication to work. The following is a list of problems you may encounter while waiting for it to kick in:

- Your hallucinations continue.
- It feels like people are talking about you.
- You think someone is going to hurt you.
- You feel like something is wrong with your body.
- Your thoughts are confused.
- You experience any of the other positive symptoms described in chapter 4.

While you wait for the symptoms to diminish:

- Be very careful to take your medicine as prescribed.
- Be sure to tell your doctor or therapist about any symptoms you experience.
- Check with someone you trust and ask him or her to help you reality test.
- Remember that you have control over what you do. You do not have to do what voices tell you to do.
- Change what you are doing when you begin to experience symptoms. For example, go for a walk, listen to music, or talk to someone.
- Tell yourself, "This is a symptom of a biological illness. It will get better."
- Remind yourself that the medicine takes time to work.
- If you feel you are losing control, contact your doctor immediately.
- If you cannot reach your doctor within a short amount of time, go to the nearest hospital emergency room or call 911.

The Fading out of Delusions: A Two-Part Gradual Process

While your brain chemicals were not functioning correctly, you most likely had many unusual thoughts. Maybe you believed people were watching you. Naturally you began to be extra-vigilant: you checked the windows an awful lot, looked around rooms for cameras or hidden microphones, suspected the phone line was tapped, and listened to every little noise. This is a good example of positive symptoms that may take time to diminish.

The way we think about things can be described as a "cognitive map." A cognitive map connects our life experiences together and helps us make decisions in the future. For example, you get stung by several bees when you sit under a tree in a park. Your brain probably stores away the connection between bees and parks so that the next time someone asks you to go on a picnic or to sit under a tree, you are reluctant. Your automatic answer is "No way." Similarly, if you are afraid people are watching you—even if it is only because of the chemical imbalance that's sending you the wrong messages—your brain stores away that automatic thought.

Once you have an "automatic thought" it is very hard to get rid of. In fact, it may lie deeply hidden in the brain's memory. As you get better with medication your thinking becomes clearer. You naturally—or sometimes with help from others—begin to question psychotic thoughts. And that is very good.

If you believed people were watching you during your psychotic period, the medication will help restore your powers to reality test so that gradually your unusual thoughts will decrease. You will stop checking out the windows, looking for cameras, listening to every sound. But do not get frightened if you find once in a while you automatically go back to your old ways—especially during moments of stress. Automatic thinking takes time and work to change.

JAMES: I did a lot of ignoring when I came out of the hospital. Most of the time when the symptoms came, it was when I wasn't taking the medicine like I should have been, every day. At first I was boldly going up to people because I thought they were talking about me, but you can't do that with everybody, so I just ignored it. When I get home from work I try to keep a hobby going, like working out or building a remote-control car.

BUDDY: Know you have to take a pill every single day. It becomes part of your life, so it becomes annoying, but I know in order to stay well and healthy I have to take it. When I stopped the Prolixin my job became stressful, and it felt like everybody was after me. It's hard coping with all these potential side effects and weight gain from the medication. Also, if the medication doesn't work, try a new medication until they find one that does the job.

JOSEPH: First thing was to realize that everything that happened was in my head, that there was no FBI following me, no video cameras in my house. The medicine played a tremendous role in helping me, but it took time, like two or three weeks, before I started to actually feel a change. Actually, at first I revolted. I thought, if I'm in here and I'm giving up marijuana, then why am I going to replace one drug with another? I said, "I'm not taking it." They told me, "If you don't take your medicine, you won't leave the hospital." That did it. I said okay.

Do not cloud your mind with marijuana. It doesn't have any effect besides clouding your mind, your goals, your judgment, dreams, and aspirations. It just wipes them out. I don't want to sound like a commercial, but it's the truth.

It took a lot of time; everything didn't happen overnight.

LAURIE: When I am quiet and I am by myself and am having bad thoughts, I tell myself to please make this thought go away. Sometimes it works and it goes away. Sometimes I hide in my room, and sometimes that helps but sometimes it doesn't. My social worker helps me. I just tell her my problems and I get feedback. Talking to my family also helps me put my fear into words. It gives me a better understanding of things.

MARCUS: Try to get out, try not to be alone, try to do something active, and, if that doesn't work, try to talk it out with your family and your doctors. I used to like to take walks, do push-ups, just to keep my mind off the problem.

AUDREY: Keep regular sleep patterns, stay away from drugs, take medicine, see your doctor, check with family members to see how they think you are doing, and be aware of your symptoms.

COPING WITH NEGATIVE SYMPTOMS

PATRICK: When I was about twenty-eight, I used to work for UPS. I was fired. From that point on my mother saw a change. I was talking to myself. If you've never been fired before, it's like a shock. I kept very much to myself, with no friends, and I never talked about my problems. Once in a while I would get angry with my parents.

They first put me on Low III, where they said clozapine would be the answer. My mother was reading in the paper that it was a good medication and helps most of the patients. So they started me on 75 milligrams and went up to 150. I stayed on Low III for three weeks. Other people's problems seemed worse, people screaming, yelling. It was a little rough, disturbing to see a lot of people walking around yelling and screaming. I felt out of place. My parents would come and I would ask them to get me out.

After three weeks I went over to day hospital. That's where I met one of my friends. I stayed there maybe six months. Then I went to my counselor and she told me about Micrographics. At Micrographics they put me in production, and later they gave me a test to see if I was up to working in the files. Then after that they got me a job.

My energy level is still low. I try to go out and exercise a little, like bike ride or walk. I met a friend, and that's helped me. I try to be more in the conversation when friends and relatives come over. I try to be talking, not to be left out. My mind gets scattered. I try to concentrate more on the subject. If you have a lot of things on your mind, try to keep an open part of your mind to deal with reality. Think about the subject so your mind doesn't wander. I have a problem with talking to myself; when my parents tell me, I try to stop it.

Accepting help from other people, especially my parents, is important.

Coping with the idea that I have this illness is also hard. When I go to group, I think mine is not so bad. It makes me think more positively about myself. Some people are doing better, but you have to be able to accept it. What else helps? Stick to your goals.

The following are some of the negative symptoms with which people often struggle and suggestions about how you can deal with them:

1. You Do Not Feel Like Doing Anything.

Having no motivation, low energy, and little enjoyment in activities is very difficult to overcome. The less you do, the less you will feel like doing. For this reason, you must work on breaking the cycle of inactivity.

- Make a list of five activities you can do when you have free time. Put the list in a noticeable place, such as on the refrigerator door. Then, when you are sitting around doing nothing, walk over to the list and choose one activity. Some sample activities we have used are walking the dog, going for a bike ride, making follow-up calls for a volunteer job, exercising for ten minutes, writing a poem, playing the guitar, and calling a specific friend.
- Build structure into your day. If you are not doing anything, take a course; find a job; volunteer; participate in a day program, a rehabilitation program, a drop-in center, or a clubhouse.
- Make plans for at least one pleasurable activity every weekend.
- Plan for daily exercise. Begin with ten minutes a day to get your motor started.

2. Your Family Says You Do Not Look Good.

Sometimes when people are not feeling well, they don't dress well or take care of their hygiene the way they did before becoming ill. This causes a problem because if you do not look well, people think there is something wrong with you. Here is a list of hints to keep you looking good.

125

- Shower daily.
- Use deodorant.
- Keep your hair clean.
- Stay clean-shaven (for males).
- Brush your teeth daily.
- Wear clean clothing.
- Take off your coat whenever you are in a heated room.

3. It's So Hard to Look at People.

For many people with schizophrenia, it is very hard to make eye contact. Some people say they feel uncomfortable. Sometimes this is due to paranoid symptoms or the worry that other people will be able to read their minds. Other times it is a habit that started long before the illness. When you are ready, begin to work on making eye contact.

Eye contact is part of how we communicate. It is almost as important as the words we speak. It lets people know we are interested in what they are saying. It builds trust. These are very important elements in socializing and working.

- Talk with your group or counselor about what it is that bothers you when you look at someone.
- Practice looking at people when you talk.
- Ask your family or friends to point out when you are not making eye contact.
- Work with your treatment group to make you aware of lapses in eye contact.

4. You Feel Tired All the Time.

Feeling tired may be a negative symptom, or it may be caused by your medicine. (See chapter 11 for a discussion of coping with side effects.) Unfortunately, there is no easy way to fill yourself with energy.

- Let your doctor know you are tired. Sometimes the doctor can add to or adjust your medications to help this problem.
- Force yourself out of bed. Place your alarm clock away from your bed so you will need to get out of bed to turn it off. Use a second clock if necessary.

- Don't get back into the bed once you are out of it.
- Exercise! Any kind of activity that gets your body moving will increase your energy.

5. It's Hard to Keep a Conversation Going.

To increase your ability to communicate, work on building your skills one step at a time. At first it will seem strange, but gradually it will come more naturally.

Step 1: Practice listening to people.

Step 2: Repeat back to them what you hear them say. Example: The person next to you says, "I am bored by my life." You say: "I heard you say you are bored."

Step 3: Add a follow-up question based on something that person said. Example: "So, why are you bored?"

Step 4: When you find yourself not knowing what to ask, remember who, what, when, where, why, and how. These are six words that will help you in most situations when you don't know what to say. Choose one to ask your question.

Make a special effort to be curious about people and things. Be a detective when you are with people. This will increase your interaction and show your interest. Practice each step for at least a week before going on to the next one. In just a few months you are likely to find it easier and fun to interact with family, friends, and new acquaintances.

> *Keys to Conversation*
> Be curious about people. Be like a reporter asking *who, what, when, where, why,* and *how* questions to keep conversations going.

AMBER: For negative symptoms, I recommend finding something you like to do, like listening to music, reading, exercising, dancing, or even watching TV. I occupy my time with things I like to do. I read magazines, dance, and exercise a few times a week. I like hanging out with friends. As for the poor concentration, I think time has helped me. When I first got sick, my concentration was not as good as it used to be. I had a hard time reading. As time went by I started reading newspapers and magazines every day. My concentration is back to normal now.

LUCINDA: The only symptom I had was tiredness. I've learned to cope with that by going to bed earlier and using three alarm clocks to wake me up in the morning.

MARK: A very important thing is mental activity. The biggest thing for me was when I couldn't think. I had a difficult time reading or playing music. But I kept trying. I think it is so important to have mental activity. If you don't use your brain, it's not going to happen. An object that is in motion has a tendency to stay in motion. That's the way I think it is in rehabilitation. It does sometimes feel like you're pushing against a wall. With enough resistance, that wall seems to move. Mental activity was the way to recovery for me, to think about something, read a book and feel something. Even to enjoy a friend you need mental activity. It can be music, art; but you need to use your cognitive mind.

THOMAS: I do things to try to take my mind off the problem, like watching TV, talking to my family. I read, listen to music, go shopping. There's not too much I can do with my tiredness. I try not to go to bed too late so I can get enough rest.

Take your medicine. Stay away from things like drugs and alcohol. Talk to the doctors. Talk to your friends and people you care about.

RICHIE: I pray. You have to push yourself to do it. If you were working out, push yourself to do that again. You just have to make yourself do it. With time, it went away for me. I remember I felt so down I didn't even want to put on my shoes. I just forced myself, and eventually I did it.

MARCUS: Don't blame yourself—that's number one. Talk to your doctors and try to get the right medication that works. Try to stay active. Try to go to school or get a job so you don't dwell on your problem. Take your medication. Try to socialize with your friends at least one day a week. Talk it out with your family or doctors.

MARK: At the beginning I was so distraught that I was having side effects or symptoms that made me feel numb. I thought, "Life isn't worth living. I'll go off the medication and go crazy." So even if you are feeling the biggest despair or self-pity, give it a little time. Complain. Try to switch your medication.

Additional resources:

Me, Myself, and Them: A Firsthand Account of One Young Person's Experience with Schizophrenia, by Kurt Snyder, Raquel E. Gur, and Linda Wasmer Andrews (Oxford University Press, 2007).

128

Getting Your Life Back Together When You Have Schizophrenia, by Roberta Temes (New Harbinger, 2002).

Schizophrenia for Dummies, by Jerome Levine and Irene S. Levine (Wiley, 2009).

COPING WITH OTHER SYMPTOMS AND SIDE EFFECTS

In addition to the positive and negative symptoms, you may also have some anxiety problems, a depressed mood, or even problems organizing your time. To make matters more complicated, the medication you take to help alleviate the symptoms of your illness often causes side effects that many people have difficulty adjusting to. In this chapter we discuss some strategies to deal with anxiety, concentration problems, and disorganization, as well as side effects such as the weight gain caused by your medication.

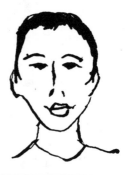

VAN

VAN: It started when I went to meet my father—I had to keep it a secret. After finally meeting him in Washington, I came back home. My mother

Special contributor: Linda Porto, R.N.

was very upset with me, and it became difficult to live with her. So I left my mother and went to live with another part of my family. I started to use drugs. I was trying to finish college and get a degree and support myself, but I became very overwhelmed and developed schizophrenia symptoms.

I was terribly frightened and realized that I needed help. I came to Hillside a few days later. I didn't know it was a hospital until a few weeks later. At first I wasn't aware of where I was, so I liked it, being with people. But when I realized the reason I was there I became upset and paranoid. I felt like I was in hiding from the authorities. I thought I had put my family in legal jeopardy. I thought I had become a media sensation like Amy Fisher. I thought I was under arrest. I realized I needed more help. Therefore I accepted the therapy and all the treatment and was receptive to the advice of the staff.

I started taking clozapine and I was thankful that small doses had a positive effect on me. I kept my treatment team informed about my trouble sleeping or being overly anxious. Just continued communicating. I would listen to other people's advice and realize that it takes time. Things aren't answered in one day and things aren't created in one day. When I get anxious, I remember those words. Breathing exercises definitely have been the thing that's helped me a lot, and exercise itself—running, aerobic, cardiovascular.

ANXIETY

Anxiety is a feeling that for some people is like butterflies in the stomach. For others it is more like fear. Anxiety affects the body in many ways, creating muscle tension, headache, shortness of breath, racing heartbeat, perspiration, and stomach upset.

Millions of years ago, humans needed anxiety just to survive day to day. It was the early warning system against dangers in the environment, which allowed humans to react almost immediately to anything that threatened their safety. Imagine if our ancestors did not have this warning system and had to stop and think through a dangerous event before acting on it: *I hear large footsteps. I feel the earth moving. Something smells bad. The birds are all quiet. What could this mean? Aha! Maybe a wild elephant is coming. I should run fast. Feet, start moving!*

A shortcut was programmed into our brains so we did not need to take the time to think about possible dangers in the environment before react-ing to them. As soon as we felt anxious, our programming (or instinct) sent us into action. We would either freeze, run, or fight.

Although there are far fewer dangers today for most people, we still feel anxiety, and it is not a good feeling. Generally, people feel anxious when they are overwhelmed by events in life or find themselves in un-comfortable situations. Many people with schizophrenia also have feel-ings of anxiety that are directly connected to the disease. Sometimes anxiety occurs because symptoms cause people to feel there is danger or to have difficulty making sense of thoughts or feelings. As people begin to feel better, they sometimes get anxious about the possibility of having symptoms again. Some people get especially anxious that they are getting sick whenever they feel any anxiety—in other words, they get anxious about feeling anxious.

Anxiety is always going to exist, so knowing how to cope with it is important. Here are some tips:

- Get to know the feelings that accompany your anxiety. Do you get fearful or queasy? Does your heart race, or do your palms sweat? Do you get headaches or muscle tension? Do you bite your nails? Do you clench your jaw?
- Tell yourself this is a signal that something is frightening you.
- Take three slow, deep breaths. Listen to your breath going in and going out.
- If possible, talk to someone about what is frightening you. If not, write it down.
- Remind yourself that your anxiety is only a feeling and it will go away.
- Take three more slow, deep breaths. Then find an activity to help you change the direction of your thoughts.

If your anxiety does not decrease, advise the people treating you.

JACKIE: I just take the medication and it goes away. I've learned some techniques to relax myself. Even now, when I'm healthy, I still do them. I breathe deeply. Sometimes I meditate.

VANESSA: I talk to my friends. I try to keep in contact with somebody.

I speak to my sister, especially my older sister, because she said anytime I need anything to just call her. I try not to think about it. I play with my kids. I just try to keep my mind off it. I try to keep myself busy.

BETH: Every time that I've gotten sick, I've had anxiety before. So when I would get anxious I would think about it and get more anxious because I'd think it was going to turn into another relapse. I have anxiety now, but I don't think I'm getting sick. I just think I have anxiety. Breathing, medication, definitely talking to people, discussing the anxiety, relaxation, and getting my mind off it are the main things for me, I think.

DISORGANIZATION

Many people find they are doing well in most ways but cannot seem to get organized. Problems include missed appointments, falling behind in work or homework assignments, and misplacing things.

Here are a few tools that will help you be organized:

Lists

Keep a list of things to do.

Number items on the list according to which ones need to be done first.

Look at the list every morning and evening.

Calendars

Enter all appointments immediately.

Write in reminders of things to do.

Look at the calendar at the same time each day.

Goal Setting

Keep a list of your long-term goals.

Keep a list of some shorter-term goals.

Setting goals can be overwhelming—break them down into small steps. Write down what the steps will be. Check off each step as you complete it.

> Example: You set a goal of going back to school.
>
> Step 1—Call three local schools for information.
>
> Step 2—Choose two schools that interest you.
>
> Step 3—Visit one of the schools.

Step 4—Visit the second school.

Step 5—Speak with a counselor about the disabilities program.

Step 6—Look at the applications.

Step 7—Fill out one application and mail it.

134

Step 8—Fill out the second application and mail it.

By taking a little piece at a time, you can work on problems that might otherwise seem impossible.

BUDDY: Try to write everything out, your daily and weekly activities. That proves effective for me, anyway. Keep a planner with appointments and scheduled dates and events. Try to be systematic, more organized.

Don't try to do too much at a time, in one day. Take one step at a time. Try to push yourself. Tell yourself you've got to do it because if you don't, it will just get worse and worse.

CONCENTRATION PROBLEMS

Your ability to concentrate will come back slowly. However, you can work on improving it. You need to let the people treating you know about your problems with concentration, which might include the following:

It's Hard to Read.

Be patient with yourself.

Begin by reading magazines.

Move on to easy, entertaining books.

Return to the type of reading you did before your illness.

It's Hard to Concentrate on Homework.

Make a schedule.

Set short-term goals for work. Plan to work for no more than one hour at a time.

Write down exactly what you hope to work on and when.

Whenever possible go to the library, away from noise and distractions.

Take notes as you read—this helps memory.

Check off completed work on your list.

Example: Marcus needs to read the assigned material for his history class.

Goal: To study one hour each weekday (from 4:00–5:00 p.m.) and one to three hours on Saturday and Sunday (11:00 a.m., 4:00 p.m., and 7:00 p.m.)

Schedule:

Monday: Read pages 1–15

Tuesday: Read pages 16–30

Wednesday: Read pages 31–45

Thursday: Read pages 46–60

Friday: Read pages 61–75

Saturday: Read pages 76–90, plus any catch-up work

Sunday: Review chapters and make notes

OTHER SYMPTOMS

Ruminating Thoughts

These are thoughts that go around and around. They get you nowhere but can keep you worried and unable to function fully. Medicine and therapy can help with this problem.

Obsessive-Compulsive Symptoms

Obsessions are thoughts that are irrational and interfere with your ability to think. Obsessive thoughts may lead to compulsive behaviors. An example is thinking that something bad will happen if you do not wash your hands repeatedly, and therefore constantly washing and rubbing your hands. Often antipsychotic medications can help with these symptoms. At other times special medication and a special type of treatment that focuses on changing behaviors may be required.

Depression

Depression is feeling down, sad, without energy, and without pleasure. You may think that life is not worth living. It is always important to get help with depression. Let the people treating you know if you are feeling depressed, because it can be helped by medication and therapy. If you are so depressed that you are thinking about killing yourself, get help immediately. Call 911 or go to the nearest emergency room.

JACKIE: There were times I used to ruminate for hours before I went to work. I made a list of things I could do when I caught myself ruminating. It took some time, but it just became second nature to get up and do something when I started ruminating. I see a therapist once a week. And I've had group therapy. It has helped me a lot.

AUDREY: About a year after my first episode I had a severe manic episode, and again I became psychotic. Following that I was put on lithium and became very depressed. I wanted to make people notice that I was depressed so I could get help. My parents were very much in denial. I reached out to them, but I didn't make myself clear. Then I took a lot of pills. I told my dad right away because what I really wanted was help. I was out of the hospital in a week.

Violent Thoughts

For some people psychotic thoughts can become very nasty. Often this happens because they believe someone is going to hurt them. They begin to have thoughts about hurting other people in order to protect themselves or simply because their thoughts make them incredibly angry. Sometimes people hear voices (auditory hallucinations) commanding them to hurt someone. For some, violent thoughts may turn to thoughts about hurting themselves.. When they recover this makes little sense, but at the time it feels very real and can lead to tragedy for the person with psychosis as well as other innocent people.

It is absolutely essential that you reach out for help if you find yourself thinking about getting a weapon or wanting to hurt yourself or someone else. Do not be afraid to spend a few days in a hospital if needed to get past violent thoughts. They can be treated.

Remember, what we think about affects how we feel and what we do. For this reason it is a good idea to stay away from violent activities. Even violent movies and violent computer games can affect thinking and behavior.

WEIGHT GAIN

Many antipsychotic medications cause weight gain. The reasons are complex, but to put it simply, medications may slow down your metabolism and increase your appetite. It is hard to lose weight and cope with medication and symptoms.

Getting Started

- You must want to lose weight.
- Identify your reasons not to gain weight (examples: looking good, having more energy, having more self-confidence, and being healthy).
- Instead of thinking of dieting, think of eating healthy.
- Find a way to make it fun.
- Choose activities that boost your metabolism and that you also enjoy (examples: swimming, running, playing ball, or dancing).

137

> *Pedometer: 10,000 Steps to Fitness*
> Walking helps you keep fit and healthy. Wear a pedometer on your hip every day to measure the number of steps you walk. Set your goal to walk at least 10,000 steps a day.

Tips on Exercise

- Move your body!
  Get a pedometer and aim to walk 10,000 steps a day.
  Take the stairs instead of the elevator.
  Walk whenever possible. Dance.
  Start slowly. Just ten minutes each day makes a difference.
- Find an exercise you like.
  Ride a bike.
  Try jogging for two weeks.
  Try martial arts or yoga.
  Join a gym.
  Contact your local YMCA.
- Aerobic exercise (getting your breathing and heart rate up) burns fat.
- Weight training builds muscle, which burns fat.
- The benefits of exercise:
  Burns fat
  Increases energy
  Increases muscle mass
  Helps your heart
  Lowers blood pressure
  Protects your bones
  Improves your mood

Just keep moving. You will find yourself feeling less tired and less hungry.

Establish Good Eating Habits

- Eat three meals a day containing "real" foods (those found naturally in nature—for example, potatoes are real; potato chips are not).
- Drink a glass of water before a meal.
- Sit down to eat.
- Chew slowly and really taste your food.
- Put your fork down between bites.
- Drink water and fruit-flavored teas.
- Eat greens—the greener the better.
- Eat what you like and enjoy what you eat.
- Avoid quick-fix energy foods like sugar-coated cereals, candies, and chocolate. These are good for short-term energy boosts, but you will end up becoming very hungry again in a very short period of time. Avoiding these foods keeps your blood sugar levels steady.
- Check labels to learn what is in your food. You will be surprised how many unexpected ingredients there are.
- Be aware that sodium and salt cause you to retain water and gain weight.

FRIENDLY AND UNFRIENDLY FOODS

Some foods can help you lose weight (friendly) and some can definitely work against you (unfriendly). Use good judgment, but if you splurge on the unfriendly variety, don't despair. Go back and try again with friendly foods.

Give yourself permission to make mistakes. If you have to have that slice of pizza, have it. Then go back to healthy eating. Remember, the key to maintaining your weight is exercising and eating right!

TABLE 11.1

FRIENDLY FOODS	UNFRIENDLY FOODS
Brown rice	Pastas

Oatmeal, grits, oat bran, other whole-grain cereals	Sugar-coated or high-fat cereals
Whole-grain bread	White bread
Egg whites	Whole eggs
Fruits (one a day)	Cakes and cookies
Potatoes	Diet foods
Water	Soda; excessive amounts of milk or juice
Air-popped popcorn	Candy
Good fats, which include poultry, low-fat cheese, nuts and seeds, olive oil, canola oil, safflower oil, small amounts of real butter	Bad fats, which include margarine, burgers, French fries, palm oil, and coconut oil

JEFF: You try to do the best you can with the side effects like the weight gain, dry mouth, and tiredness. I'm in a weight management group. They teach you to eat healthier, drink a lot of water, and stuff like that so you can try to lose some weight.

BETH: The worst thing was I gained seventy-five pounds. That time I had off I was lazy. I stopped exercising and was eating whatever I wanted to eat. I slept for days, till five at night. The laziness, the tiredness, and the weight gain. . . . Now that it happened to me a second time, I know that the medicine really causes the weight gain. But I think if you are conscious of it you can do things about it.

METABOLIC AND CARDIOVASCULAR SIDE EFFECTS

The newer antipsychotic medications can cause metabolic and cardiovascular problems for many people. The metabolic effects include weight gain, increased cholesterol, and increased insulin levels. This increases the risk of diabetes and heart problems. For this reason it is very important to see your medical doctor every six months or sooner if you have signs of heart or diabetes problems. You may ask your psychiatrist if it is possible to change your antipsychotic medication to one with fewer metabolic effects, but do not be disappointed if he or she does not believe that is a good idea for you. The psychiatrist's decision depends on which medications work best for your psychosis. Sometimes doctors will prescribe medicine such as metformin (Glucophage) to help you stop gaining or lose weight. A good diet and exercise plan can make a big difference in keeping your weight down and health problems in check. *Never take an over-the-counter weight-loss drug because many of them have ingredients that may increase the risk for psychosis.*

OTHER SIDE EFFECTS

Most side effects are caused by medication. For this reason, you usually must decide which are worse: the psychotic symptoms or the side effects you are experiencing. Almost always the answer is that the psychotic symptoms are worse. And often side effects such as stiffness and tremors can be decreased by working with your doctor to adjust your medication, change it if necessary, or add another medication that works specifically to counteract a particular side effect.

In addition, many side effects diminish over time. Tiredness generally goes away as your body adjusts to the medication. Drooling also gets better with time. Even the increased appetite may level off after several months.

Additional resources:

The National Institute of Mental Health book on schizophrenia has a section on side effects of medications: http://www.nimh.nih.gov/health/publications/schizophrenia/index.shtml

Schizophrenia.com: www.schizophrenia.com/family.php

12 DRUGS, ALCOHOL, AND SAFER SEX

Drugs, alcohol, and safe sex are important topics for everyone to understand. If you already have a drug or alcohol problem, then you need to know how this can affect your schizophrenia and what you can do to eliminate drugs and alcohol from your life. If you do not have a problem, then knowing the facts can keep you from developing one. Knowing how to prevent sexually transmitted diseases is also important because these illnesses can add lots of stress to your life.

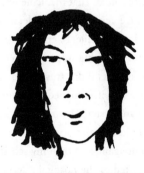

RICHIE

RICHIE: When I was nineteen I was in high school. I was hanging out with the wrong crowd, smoking marijuana. When I was high I would think about having AIDS. I thought I was Jesus. I thought that the whole

Special contributor: Alan Mendelowitz, M.D.

world knew me—I thought I was famous. Remember that movie with Jim Carrey, *The Truman Show*, where everybody was watching him on TV? That was the same way I felt. Maybe they got that story from somebody with schizophrenia. I thought I was psychic, that I could control people, put things into people's heads. I remember all these things when I was smoking, like people were after me—paranoia.

Then later, after the high went away, the thoughts stayed with me. I would think the radio was giving me messages, that the artists would be in the studio singing the songs just to me. I thought there was a camera in the TV watching me. I was playing music real loud and I didn't want to stop. Then I started breaking things in my room—I pulled the door off the hinges.

My mother got scared and she called the cops on me. Then the cops took me to St. John's Hospital. They shot me with a needle so I could calm down and relax. The next day I was having visions. On the way home from the hospital I was looking at the cab driver, and it looked like his hand was on fire. So then they brought me to Zucker Hillside Hospital and they put me in Low III.

They put me on a medicine called clozapine. But the medicine was making me too sleepy. When I went back to school I would fall asleep. A few weeks after I got out of the hospital, I stopped taking the medicine. Then they put me on Risperdal. That medicine was making me feel slow, and I would drool a lot. I felt uncomfortable, so I stopped taking that one too. I didn't get sick for a while. I kept it a secret that I wasn't taking the medicine. The doctor knew. He was trying to tell me I would get sick again, but I didn't believe him. I didn't trust him. I figured it was the marijuana that made me sick and if I stopped smoking I would be okay. So I dropped out of school and I started working in a gym. That was in the beginning of the year. I did well all the way to Thanksgiving, almost a year.

I started smoking pot again, and then my schizophrenia started kicking in again. I got admitted to the hospital a second time. That's when I was introduced to olanzapine. The only problem with that was it made me gain weight. I didn't like being heavy, so I stopped taking the medicine again. I started working with my uncle and going to school to get my GED. I started having delusions again. I felt like life wasn't real, like it was fake or something. I thought I was getting messages out of cartoons, like the Spiderman cartoons. Then I went back to the hospital again for a week. I think they let me out early because I had a job at a grocery store.

I got admitted to the hospital again when I stopped my medicine another time because I didn't want to gain weight. While I was in the hospital my mother came to visit me. When she was at the door, ready to leave, I made believe I was going to get money from her. Then I just ran out the door. I had six dollars in my pocket. I ran to the bus. I took the bus to Kew Gardens and the F train to Manhattan. I remember it was kind of cold and all I had on was a T-shirt. I walked around Manhattan and got on the A train to go home. The next two days I stayed home. Then my father took me to see Mrs. Miller at the hospital so I could fill out some papers. Before I knew it, five guys carried me back into Low III. That's when I started taking Haldol. I was in the hospital for a month, and since I started taking Haldol I've been out of the hospital for a year straight. I've been in the hospital for a total of six times because I stopped taking my medicine. Now I've been taking it consistently, and I haven't been back into the hospital and I haven't had any delusions or voices or paranoia.

Don't abuse drugs. You can drink occasionally, but don't do it every day. Stay away from marijuana because usually they add drugs to make it more potent so you will come back for more. But it really messes you up in the long run.

DRUGS AND ALCOHOL

Substance Abuse and People with Schizophrenia

People with schizophrenia have a higher rate of substance abuse than people who do not have schizophrenia. There have been many theories about why people with schizophrenia use substances. Over the years, one of the most popular has been the self-medication hypothesis. This theory suggests that as people become ill and have frightening thoughts and hallucinations, they look for substances in order to treat themselves. Though this applies to some people, it does not apply to everyone. Another theory is that there is a chemical imbalance in the brain related to the chemical imbalance that causes schizophrenia. These imbalances may increase the likelihood that a person with schizophrenia will become involved with drugs and alcohol. It is possible that the brain's mechanism of reinforcing addictive behaviors involves the same transmitters that we believe are partly responsible for causing psychotic symptoms.

Theories Linking Schizophrenia with Substance Abuse
People with schizophrenia use drugs and alcohol in order to self-medicate.
Alcohol and drug abuse may also be caused by an imbalance of neurotransmitters. This imbalance may trigger a chemical reaction that sends out messages demanding more of those substances.

GARY: It's not a good idea for those who have had the illness to take drugs because we are especially sensitive.

BEN: Obviously drugs alter your state of thinking. They just totally don't mix with prescription drugs. The same with alcohol. It screws up your chemistry.

Genetics, Environment, and Peer Group

There are many factors that determine which people with schizophrenia become involved with drugs and alcohol. The three major risk factors are *genetics*, the *environment*, and the *peer group* with whom you spend time.

The genetic risk involves the genes people inherit that may put them at risk for a chemical imbalance that reinforces the use of substances. The environment in which one is brought up—including parents, siblings, and family system—may also contribute to alcohol and drug use. Perhaps the risk factor that people have the most control over is the peer group they join and the friends that they spend time with. It is more likely that if your friends smoke, drink, and use drugs, you will. It is important to encourage your friends not to use drugs and alcohol. If you can't, try to find the strength to make a new set of friends, because these substances are harmful to you.

AMBER: I don't take drugs. When I'm out with friends I try not to drink alcohol. Sometimes I feel some pressure when I go out with my friends, but I stop and think and remind myself that I am on medication. I just order a cranberry juice or water instead.

JEFF: I know that I am on the drug olanzapine. Once in a while I'll have a beer on a weekend. Not very often. I know you are not supposed to, but I do anyway.

SMOKEY: I got in more trouble when I drank. Don't drink and don't smoke weed. Most people get sicker.

RECENT FINDINGS ON DRUG AND ALCOHOL USE

- Having schizophrenia increases your chance of having an alcohol problem 10 times.
- Having schizophrenia increases your chance of having a drug problem 7.6 times.
- The lifetime risk of a person with schizophrenia for alcohol or drug problems is almost 50 percent.
- People who have schizophrenia are 4 to 5 times more likely to smoke cigarettes than other people.
- Nicotine and caffeine are the two drugs used most often by people with schizophrenia.

Do Substances Cause Schizophrenia?

LAURIE: I believe drugs and alcohol are the reason I am sick today.

Many years ago people thought that drug abuse was one of the causes of schizophrenia. Over the years we have learned that drugs can contribute to symptoms of psychosis, but for most people drug use does not appear to cause a long-standing illness such as schizophrenia. For example, daily use of marijuana can bring on paranoia and negative symptoms, but for many people those symptoms will disappear within a few weeks of stopping marijuana use. Nevertheless, there is evidence that people who use marijuana develop schizophrenia at an earlier age than those who don't use marijuana and a new concern that daily users run a risk of developing a schizophrenia type of illness. It is also possible that PCP use by an individual at risk will bring on psychotic symptoms of schizophrenia earlier than they might have appeared otherwise.

The Effect of Drugs and Alcohol on Psychotic Symptoms

It is known that street drugs can contribute to a worsening of symptoms even when someone is taking their medication. We also know substance-abusing people with schizophrenia are more likely to become ill at a younger age, have lower rates of adhering to treatment, and usually do not function as well as people with schizophrenia who do not have a substance abuse problem.

Each drug affects people in its own unique way. A psychosis caused by the use of stimulants or cocaine looks more like mania (bipolar disorder) than schizophrenia. The symptoms include hyperactivity, racing thoughts, pressured speech, and paranoid ideas. They usually do not include other symptoms of schizophrenia, such as hallucinations or negative symptoms. Hallucinogens, such as LSD, can cause a psychosis that usually involves visual and tactile hallucinations. Acute intoxication with PCP or ecstasy most resembles schizophrenia. Marijuana, used by many people before their first psychotic break, can also lead to an increase of paranoid delusions and referential thinking.

Alcohol is one drug about which it is difficult to draw conclusions. Alcohol is initially relaxing, but then it brings on depressive symptoms, which can be very distressing. The results of an acute alcohol binge can look the same as a psychotic relapse. Alcohol withdrawal can sometimes be severe and cause psychosis. This is called delirium tremens, or d.t.'s.

BETH: When I came out of the hospital the first time and went back to school a year after my episode, I drank and smoked pot like a regular college student. I did it while I was taking my medication, and then I wound up getting sick. Since my relapse I haven't used alcohol or smoked because I am afraid. I would rather be healthy than be drunk. But I am not happy about it because I miss being drunk and I miss being high. I go to the bars all the time and I watch my friends drink, and it's difficult.

JAMES: Man, that put me in a time warp—it took me back to when I was first feeling symptoms and using marijuana. That was a dumb thing. I wouldn't advise anybody to use drugs. I wouldn't want anybody to feel those symptoms. The same symptoms from when you first got into the hospital are going to come right back to you. You are going to get scared. I ended right back in the emergency room.

SHARON: Stay away from that garbage. It is just going to make you paranoid. I just felt like I wasn't real and I became hypersexual.

VAN: I think something not to do is use drugs to try to help yourself, because it doesn't help. It will bring you to a lower state, which is more difficult to recover from. It can be very dangerous in your recovery and not a positive choice. I know because I have experienced it.

Chronic Alcohol Use

Daily or chronic alcohol use has serious medical implications, including potential liver damage and cirrhosis, as well as an adverse effect on the

146

metabolism. It decreases the liver's ability to metabolize medications. This is important because the medications make it possible to effectively treat symptoms.

One of the severe dangers associated with chronic alcohol use is the potential for withdrawal reactions. These can range from mild to severe and life threatening. A mild withdrawal reaction might involve having the shakes, craving a morning drink, and feeling miserable for a few days. Chronic use can put people at risk for more severe reactions including seizures and, in the worst case scenario, d.t.'s (delirium tremens). D.t.'s often occur about five days after someone has stopped long-term daily alcohol use. They can include many psychiatric symptoms and can look the same as a psychotic relapse. As this is a dangerous withdrawal syndrome, it must be treated medically in the hospital.

147

As a rule, we recommend abstinence from alcohol. Our clinical experience has been that for most people, alcohol use has negative consequences.

MARCUS: Stay away from alcohol because it won't mix with the medication. I used to drink a lot with my friends. It's been two years now that I've been sober, and I don't have any temptations at all, none at all.

Do You Have a Problem with Alcohol?

Ask yourself the following questions. If you say "yes" to more than one, talk to the people who are treating you about the fact that you might have a problem with alcohol.

1. Do you drink every day?
2. Do you drink first thing in the morning?
3. Do you drink alone, when you are not in social situations?
4. If you don't drink for two or three days, do you get the shakes?
5. Does drinking interfere with your life and relationships?

ZELDA: I think I used alcohol as a tool to sort of bring out my outgoing personality and be a little less concentrated on my fears. I had to learn how to live without that shield. And it's very tempting because the world goes on presenting alcohol to you. You just have to remember that it's not going to save you. It will only make things worse in the long run.

MEREDITH: Don't let other people make you feel like you're missing something because you're not drinking with them. It's hard when you're in a drinking or drug environment and you say, "Coke" (as in cola) and they say, "Coke?" (as in cocaine).

148

Treatment for Schizophrenia and Drug/Alcohol Dependence

There are no safe street drugs for people who have schizophrenia. Problems with alcohol and drugs affect up to 50 percent of people with schizophrenia. Since these problems can contribute to symptoms, handling them must be part of the treatment plan.

Initially it is very difficult to give up alcohol or drugs when you have become addicted. First you have to admit that you have a problem. Next you will need the courage to face that you need help. Then you can begin building your motivation to be abstinent. All this before you begin to set out a plan for stopping your drug or alcohol use.

The best and easiest way to beat your addiction is to be involved in a dual diagnosis program that can focus on both psychiatric symptoms and symptoms of substance abuse. Structured programs with specialized staff often use a supportive AA model to help people maintain their abstinence and sobriety. Dual diagnosis programs of this type are often now called MICA programs, which stands for "mentally ill chemical abuser." There are programs of all levels, dependent on the drugs to which you are addicted, the effect of your addiction on your mental and physical health, and your past efforts to stop using. These programs range from outpatient groups to day programs to inpatient treatment. Treatment can positively change the course of your schizophrenia and your life.

If you stop drinking, you must tell your physician so she or he can monitor you for withdrawal. For caffeine and nicotine, we also recommend abstinence. At the very least, discuss the use of these drugs with the people involved in your treatment.

Cigarette Smoking

So what about smoking? Everyone seems to be doing it, even when people say it is bad for you. What exactly is the problem with cigarettes?

Unlike other descriptions you may have heard of smoking as all bad, here are some good things about smoking. We'll get to the bad later.

It sharpens the way I think: There is evidence that shows that smoking may temporarily improve cognition, the thinking process and focusing. This is because nicotine binds with receptors in the brain that act positively on the ability to concentrate and think logically. Researchers have shown that people are better able to ignore distractions such as music in another room or loud noises in the environment when they smoke. If all of this is true, what is so bad about smoking? Many things, and that is discussed later, but even the good part is not so good. The good effects of smoking do not last very long. The receptors in the brain stop bringing about the good effects after a while. To make up for this loss, people try smoking more and more and become addicted to nicotine. With the increase in the number of cigarettes smoked the bad side effects kick in.

It makes me feel good: It is true that smoking can make you feel good, especially when you are in social situations. It does have a calming effect for many people, and some have reported feeling more relaxed when smoking. It may also reduce some of the stiffness or unwanted movements that your medications may be causing. Smoking is also a way to keep busy and feel less bored and anxious. When people who have schizophrenia were asked why they smoke, they listed all of the above reasons including that it was something they did out of habit. Of course if you are addicted to cigarettes, smoking becomes more than a social habit. It is an addiction that makes you want to smoke more to fight off the bad feeling of craving for nicotine.

Everyone smokes: It may seem that everyone you know smokes. That is because about 85 to 90 percent of people who have schizophrenia really do smoke, compared to about 25 to 30 percent of people who do not have schizophrenia. Why do more people with schizophrenia smoke when compared to everyone else? No one knows for sure, but there has been a great deal of speculation. There may be a special connection between the biology of schizophrenia, specifically the genetic makeup, and the need for nicotine. Another thought is that it has to do with releasing dopamine into the brain in a way that lessens some types of symptoms such as problems with concentration, voices, or unwanted thoughts. This is probably not true for most people, but smoking may reduce symptoms for some.

The not-so-good effects of smoking: Smoking is linked with a variety of illnesses, including cancer, heart disease, emphysema and certain types of eye diseases, just to name a few. On the average, people who smoke even 10 cigarettes a day reduce their life expectancy by two to three years. If they smoke 20 cigarettes a day they lose five to seven years, and with 40 cigarettes, eight to 10 years. If you quit, within 10 years your health risk falls to about the same as if you had never smoked. Aside from these grim statistics, smoking causes teeth to turn yellow and even increases the likelihood of getting premature wrinkles. None of these is good, but you have probably already heard people tell you that smoking is bad for you. If you still smoke there are likely two reasons: it is hard to stop or you like to smoke. There may be others, but those are the most popular.

It is hard to stop: This is true. Nicotine addiction is tough, and some people have a harder time quitting than others. There is no way to tell in advance if you will have an easier or harder time stopping, but there are ways to help you stop. You need to discuss this with your doctor because certain prescription medications and patches have been shown to work. You probably should not try to stop on your own, because sometimes when people try to stop their symptoms may become more noticeable. This is usually just temporary, but your doctor can help you control symptoms if this happens to you. Also, the nicotine patch and nicotine gum must be used carefully and monitored when you are on other medications. Your doctor can guide you to make stopping easier and without harm to you. You also may have the opportunity to join a group for support. It is good to stop, and you can get the support you need from your doctor, who will be glad to help.

"I like to smoke": Millions of people feel this way, so you are not alone. Smoking is a choice, and it is yours to make as long as you know the risks that are involved. There are things that you need to remember if you smoke. Not everyone likes it. Some people may be allergic to smoke, or they may have asthma or some other problem with breathing. They may not want smoke around them. Smoke can irritate the eyes of some contact lens wearers and it is definitely bad for little children, especially babies, to be exposed to smoke. If you are in someone's home, you need to ask permission to smoke. Many people will say no or they will ask you to step outside. It is their right to want their home smoke free, and you need to understand and comply.

Important: Do not take it personally when you are asked not to smoke or to smoke elsewhere. People may have health reasons that they are not sharing with you.

Important: There are rules in some public places, such as restaurants, elevators, trains, buses, and other places. Obey the rules. Find out where you are allowed to smoke and where smoking is not permitted. Often there are signs, no smoking signs. The rules against smoking are there for reasons of health. If you are in an elevator with someone who has asthma and you light up, that person can get an attack. Secondary smoke, smoke from other people's cigarettes, can make people sick. So be a good sport and be considerate of others.

Why are cigarettes so expensive? Cigarettes are expensive—in some places close to $10 a pack—because the government places high taxes on them. These taxes are partly to discourage smoking and partly to help pay for health costs related to cigarette use. Smoking is a public health risk. People who smoke and people exposed to secondhand smoke can get sick, which means costly treatments that are often paid for by our government. This should tell you something about the high risks of smoking. Even if you are young, there is no way to tell if or when smoking will harm you. Talk it over with your doctor, nurse, or social worker. Talking doesn't mean you have to quit, but it is a good way to get started on making the right choice for you.

And, just for your information, chewing tobacco is not good for you either.

Stopping Marijuana, Alcohol, and Other Drug Use—Most People Can't Do It Themselves

Besides nicotine and caffeine, marijuana and alcohol are the two drugs most often used. But there are many other drugs as well.

We know that drugs affect the brain chemistry so that people have more symptoms of schizophrenia. This is clearly not good! Even though you might understand this, you may discover that it is very hard to stop using drugs—even marijuana—on your own. This is true for people who don't have schizophrenia too. For this reason it is important to ask for or accept help with your drug or alcohol problem.

Quitting is a process. Denying you have a problem may go on for a long time. You may require time to work on your denial and to think about all the reasons you want to stop. Then you will need to make a commitment to stop, set a stop time, and make a plan. The plan will include:

    1. understanding what triggers you to want to use

2. what you can do to eliminate, avoid, or cope with those triggers

3. holding onto your motivation to stay off the drugs or alcohol

4. a plan for getting back into your program if you do use again.

In treatment you will learn to recognize what thoughts or events act as triggers that lead to your use. And you will learn to look at the consequences. There are so many triggers around us and it is unbelievably hard to hold onto motivation when you are dealing with schizophrenia. For this reason, everyone does better when they have a group or individual counselor to help with drug use. Don't wait! If you were using drugs or alcohol before you got sick, get help to prevent your using again. If you started again after you got sick, get help to stop.

How Thoughts and Feelings Can Trigger Use of Drugs or Alcohol

Mike is lying in bed feeling angry that he has schizophrenia. He feels like a failure. He thinks, "What's the difference, I have schizophrenia anyway." Mike goes into his closet and finds some of his old marijuana and smokes it. He does not feel any difference, but he goes back to bed and skips school that day.

The THOUGHTS that triggered Mike's use were, "What's the difference, I have schizophrenia anyway."

The FEELINGS that triggered Mike's use were hopelessness and anger.

The BEHAVIOR the thoughts and feelings triggered was that he skipped school.

The CONSEQUENCE was that his parents were angry and he missed some important work he needed to learn for his finals. And he admits, he did start to have that confused, paranoid feeling again.

If Mike continues in this way he will fail out of school, feel worse about himself, have more psychotic symptoms, and not do nearly as well as he could have in his recovery from schizophrenia.

STOPPING DRUG AND ALCOHOL USE REQUIRES HELP

- Since all street drugs affect the brain in ways that worsen symptoms of schizophrenia, we strongly recommend abstinence from *all* street drugs.
- Find a treatment program that understands both schizophrenia and substance abuse issues.

- Go to AA and NA meetings with a friend so you are more comfortable.

GUIDE TO SUBSTANCES OF ABUSE

Alcohol

Alcohol can relieve anxiety and decrease depression. Unfortunately, these benefits are temporary. This is an addictive substance that can have an immediate negative effect on the liver and decrease its ability to metabolize medication. Alcohol can also cause increased depression. Binge drinking can result in symptoms that look the same as psychosis. Chronic alcohol use can result in liver damage and mild to severe withdrawal reactions.

Caffeine

Caffeine is one of the most commonly used substances in our society. It has both stimulant and addictive properties. In sensitive people it can provoke symptoms of psychosis or mania. In addition, caffeine interferes with the sleep cycle, which is very important to maintaining good psychiatric health.

We recommend that caffeine intake—which includes coffee, tea, cola products, and even chocolate—be limited for people with schizophrenia. Try to keep daily intake at 60 mg. or less.

CAFFEINE GUIDELINES
Cup of coffee—60 mg.
Cup of tea—approximately 40 mg.
Can of cola—approximately 20 mg.
Chocolate candy bar—approximately 5 mg.

Club Drugs

Club drugs are often used at dance clubs, all-night parties (sometimes known as raves and trances), and rock concerts. They give the illusion of providing extra energy, and intoxicating highs. They are most often used by young people who want to feel "deep experiences." In fact, they are quite dangerous and can cause serious brain damage and even death. When mixed with alcohol, as they often are at these events, they become even more dangerous. Examples of club drugs are MDMA (ecstasy, Adam, XTC), Rohyphnol (rohies, roofies, roach, and rope), GHB (liquid ecstasy, somatomox, scoop, Georgia home boy, and grievous bodily harm), and ketamine (special k). Ketamine is a new synthetic drug that causes hallucinations and gives people the sensation of having an out-of-body experience. It has been misused and abused in city bars as a "date rape" drug. So be very careful when you are drinking in public.

154

Sometimes young people experiment with these drugs or even mix them with alcohol. This can be extremely dangerous and can cause symptoms like depression, confusion, severe anxiety, and paranoia. Physical symptoms include muscle tension, involuntary teeth clenching, blurred vision, and increased heart rate and blood pressure.

Cocaine and Crack

When this addictive drug is sniffed, snorted, or injected, it is known as cocaine. When it is smoked, it is known as crack. Both versions are harmful in that they increase heart rate and blood pressure and can cause sudden death. When either is mixed with alcohol, the danger of sudden death increases. Cocaine and crack also can cause paranoia, aggression, and depression. Cocaine does not have a physical withdrawal syndrome, but there is very severe psychological withdrawal, including tremendous drug cravings.

Crack, the form of cocaine that is smoked, is a solid version of cocaine that looks like small rocks. It is the most addictive form of cocaine because it enters the body very fast and provides a quick high. Crack also requires less processing, and it is relatively cheap. The more a person uses it, the more addictive it becomes. People with psychosis should avoid all forms of cocaine, including crack, because it may produce intense paranoia.

Heroin

Heroin is a highly addictive drug similar to morphine; both are derived from opium. Typically, heroin is injected and brings about a fast high. It also leads to an intense, uncomfortable withdrawal. It is so addictive, it makes users want to continuously seek it out to prevent withdrawal, and they often devote their whole lives to finding the next "fix." Though some people report an initial relief of symptoms from their first experience with this drug, it is highly addictive. There is also a strong association between heroin use and involvement in criminal activity. One of the greatest dangers of using heroin is the potential for a lethal overdose. Another important danger is the risk of HIV and hepatitis when needles are shared with other people.

Inhalants

Everyday household products may be abused as inhalants. Some people experience highs from inhaling glue, paint thinners, and the propellants in aerosol cans such as deodorant sprays or whipped cream dispensers, but they are actually poisoning themselves. Using inhalants can cause irreversible damage such as hearing loss, arm and leg spasms, and brain damage. It can also harm the blood, liver, and kidneys. If used in a high concentration, inhalants can even cause death. These products are safe to use for their intended purposes, but you should always read the label for special instructions, such as only using paint thinners in a well-ventilated room.

Intravenous Drugs

Intravenous drugs are injected into the body. The most popular of these are heroin, cocaine, and "speedballing" (heroin and cocaine together). Intravenous drugs pose several additional problems. Perhaps the biggest is the increased risk of developing hepatitis B and C or the virus that causes AIDS from sharing needles with people who have already been exposed to HIV or the hepatitis virus. Sharing of needles should always be avoided.

LSD

LSD, the old '60s drug, is making a comeback. It is usually called "acid," and taking it is referred to as a "trip." Often, instead of the expected high, users experience increased heart rate and blood pressure, dilated pupils, sweating, sleeplessness, dry mouth, and tremors. Sometimes they have flashbacks to past experiences; this can be very frightening, especially when the experiences are not happy ones. It is essential to avoid this drug because there is a good probability of it making you feel very sick and emotionally upset.

Marijuana

Some people think that marijuana is okay to use and that it will do no

harm. This is not true: it can cause many unpleasant and even dangerous symptoms. Marijuana can cause memory loss, distorted perception,
thought disorders, anxiety, and even panic attacks. It can also damage the
lungs. When mixed with cocaine, it raises blood pressure and can cause
156   severe heart problems. It is not a good idea to mix marijuana with alcohol either, because the effects are unpredictable. Driving while using
marijuana is dangerous because it affects the way people see distances and
sometimes causes them to take risks. As with most drugs, taking marijuana while on medications can be especially harmful because it can produce
unexpected side effects.

Nicotine

Nicotine is one of the substances most widely used by people with schizophrenia. Like caffeine, it has both stimulant and addictive properties. It
has also been shown to have antianxiety properties. There is some evidence that it is especially difficult for people with schizophrenia or depression to give up nicotine, but this varies from person to person.

Smoking tobacco makes your liver work faster and, as a result, will
decrease the blood levels of many of the medications that we use to treat
psychotic symptoms. Nicotine has some antipsychotic and antianxiety
properties that may briefly make you feel better, but the medical risks
of cigarette smoking far outweigh its benefits. Because of its stimulant
properties and its effect on the metabolism of psychiatric medications, we
recommend abstinence from nicotine. However, we do not recommend
attempting to give up nicotine during an acute episode of illness.

Steroids, PCP, and Methamphetamine

Steroids are male sex hormones that are used by some people to build
muscle mass. They are often used illegally by athletes and body build-
ers and can produce unpleasant and even serious side effects. For men,
these can include reduced sperm count, shrinking of the testicles, baldness, development of breasts, and even increased risk of prostate cancer.
For women, side effects can include facial hair, baldness, changes in the
menstrual cycle, enlargement of the clitoris, and lowered voice. Steroids
can also cause people of both sexes to be overly aggressive and experience
severe mood swings (especially depression), paranoia, delusions, and irritability.

PCP is also known as "angel dust," "ozone," "wack," and "rocket fuel." When combined with marijuana, it is called "killer joints" and "crystal supergrass." It can be dissolved in alcohol or water, taken in pill form, or smoked. Symptoms from taking PCP may include delusions, paranoia, disordered thinking, dissociation, and catatonia. It can also make people violent and suicidal. This is a drug to be avoided.

Methamphetamine is sometimes known as "speed," "meth," or "chalk," and can be taken orally, by snorting, and by injection. The version that can be smoked is called "ice," "crystal," and "glass." Methamphetamine damages the dopamine and serotonin neurotransmitter systems, so it can cause movement disorders, strokes, and heart problems. Other side effects include irritability, insomnia, confusion, anxiety, paranoia, and aggressiveness. Methamphetamine use also can result in convulsions and death, so stay away!

Ritalin and Pain Medications

Ritalin is often prescribed to children for attention deficit-hyperactivity disorder or ADHD. It is a stimulant that can help people with ADHD but has unknown effects on those without this problem. Sometimes people abuse Ritalin by taking too much, but more often they "borrow" someone else's pills, usually those of a little brother or sister. When it is mixed with alcohol or used with cocaine, Ritalin is especially dangerous. Even alone, its effects are unpredictable, and it may exacerbate psychosis.

Pain medications prescribed to one family member are sometimes abused by others in the family. These medications should be avoided. They can be dangerous if too much is taken, and some are highly addictive. Examples include Demerol, morphine, codeine, OxyContin, and fentanyl. Common combinations of these drugs with aspirins and Tylenol have names like Darvon, Percodan, and Percocet. Unless you have a prescription and are under your doctor's orders to take them, stay away. (Source: National Institute on Drug Abuse, National Institutes of Health. Bethesda, MD. NIDA INFOFAX, www.drugabuse.gov.)

Additional resources:

http://www.cdc.gov/tobacco/data_statistics/sgr/sgr_2004/00_pdfs/SGRreportSpanish1odec04.pdf

http://www.cdc.gov/tobacco/quit_smoking/

http://www.cancer.gov/cancertopics/factsheet/Tobacco/cessation

http://www.cdc.gov/tobacco/data_statistics/sgr/sgr_2004/00_pdfs/whatitmeanstoyou.pdf

(Spanish): http://www.cdc.gov/tobacco/data_statistics/sgr/sgr_2004/00_pdfs/SGRreportSpanish10dec04.pdf

158

SAFER SEX

Sex is an important part of life. However, it is absolutely necessary to be cautious and prevent any exposure to sexually transmitted diseases. This means using condoms (a new condom for each ejaculation) for vaginal, anal, and oral sex. When you are having symptoms of psychosis, you may want to hold off on sex until you feel more like yourself. When you feel well, you may not make the same choices as you would when very ill.

There is an array of viruses that can be transmitted through the exchange of body fluids. These viruses can be dangerous to your health. By simply using the appropriate precautions, you can dramatically reduce the chances of catching a sexually transmitted disease.

STDs (Sexually Transmitted Diseases)

STD stands for sexually transmitted disease. Examples are syphilis, gonorrhea, and genital herpes. As the name indicates, it is a disease (virus) that is transmitted through unprotected sex. If one partner already has a virus, it is likely that the other partner will become infected as well, *if there was an exchange of body fluids.* Because symptoms often take a while to develop and often go unnoticed, it is next to impossible to be sure if your partner has a virus or not. Therefore, the very best prevention is to avoid having unprotected sex by always using a condom.

Hepatitis B

Similar to HIV, hepatitis B is a virus that is transmitted through the exchange of blood and other body fluids. It can be transmitted through unprotected sex, sharing of needles, and blood transfusion. Similar to HIV, it can also be passed from an infected mother to an unborn child. However, in the case of hepatitis B, there is a vaccine available. Although unprotected sex and sharing needles are never good ideas, it is highly recommended that you take further protection and get vaccinated, if you have not done so already. Also, if you have a child, make sure he or she has been vaccinated as well. Ask your doctor for further information.

Human Papillomavirus (HPV)

Cervical cancer is caused by a virus in the uterus (connected to the vagina) called human papillomavirus or HPV. HPV is a simple virus, but if it is undetected and untreated it can develop into cervical cancer. The good news is that there is a new vaccine that protects against the development of most cancer-causing HPV viruses. It is a good idea for females to get vaccinated for extra protection. It is recommended that the vaccine be administered around the age of eleven or twelve. Ask your doctor for more information.

HIV/AIDS

WHAT YOU NEED TO KNOW There are many things to know about HIV and AIDS. Here are the essentials, but if you want to learn more you can read up on the subject. At the end of this section is a list of resources that will provide more details.

WHAT ARE HIV AND AIDS? HIV (human immunodeficienty virus) is the name of a virus that causes the disease known as AIDS (acquired immunodeficiency syndrome). AIDS makes people very sick, but today there are medications to treat it. This is important to know because many people assume that AIDS always ends in death within a few years. Yes, AIDS is serious and some people do die from it, but if the disease is caught early enough, many people can live productive lives on the new medications.

HIV is called AIDS when the immune system becomes seriously damaged. This means a person technically can have the HIV virus but not AIDS. Until HIV becomes AIDS, people may have no symptoms or only a few symptoms. To lessen the confusion about this, we will just use the term HIV to refer to the disease, with or without symptoms. If a person has the virus in their system, then they are HIV positive. If a person does not have the virus in their system, then they are HIV negative.

- HIV is caused by a virus.
- "HIV positive" means a person has the HIV virus.
- "HIV negative" means a person does not have the HIV virus.
- You can be HIV positive and have few or no symptoms.
- HIV can develop into AIDS, a life-threatening illness.

- Today, with treatment, you can be HIV positive and live a productive life.

HOW DOES A PERSON CATCH HIV? HIV is contagious, but only through the exchange of body fluids. The virus is transmitted from person to person through unprotected sex, sharing dirty needles when using drugs, and accidents such as needle sticks. HIV can be transmitted from an infected mother to her unborn child and later through breast feeding. Deep kissing is another way to get HIV, although this is less common. Blood transfusions have also resulted in the transmission of HIV. You cannot get HIV by shaking hands or by sharing pens or clothing, and certainly not from being in the same room with a person who has it.

Unprotected sex, both heterosexual and homosexual, puts people at risk for HIV. Condoms are good protection, but *they must be used correctly.* Also, only latex or polyurethane condoms provide protection. Lambskin or any other type of condom will not do the job. Oral sex can also place a person at risk. Be careful. Use protection. A latex condom is the way to have safe sex. Of course, no sex is the best protection. It is wise to wait until you feel in control of your thoughts and feelings before having a sexual relationship.

Injecting drugs with dirty needles is another way of getting HIV. If you ever use drugs—which we do not recommend—use a new needle. Do not attempt to sterilize needles. It is too easy to make a mistake and the risks are too great. The best way to avoid this problem is not to use injectable drugs. You can rest easy knowing that when your doctor or nurse gives you an injection, they always use a new, disposable needle. Never try to retrieve needles out of waste cans. This is a very dangerous practice and can result in a needle stick, another way HIV is transmitted.

HOW TO PROTECT YOURSELF FROM HIV/AIDS AND OTHER STDS

- Use latex or polyurethane condoms whenever having sexual relations (anal, oral, or vaginal sex). Be sure to apply the condom correctly.
- Do not use lubricants made of petroleum products (such as Vaseline or baby oil) because petroleum breaks down the protective

properties of latex.
- Abstain from sexual relations.
- Do not share needles.

What About Testing for HIV?

If you or your doctor thinks you are at risk for getting HIV, then it is a good idea to get tested. HIV blood tests can be arranged by any health care professional, including doctors, nurses, social workers, and rehabilitation counselors, if you request it. You must agree to be tested. Routine blood tests for medications and other medical reasons do not include HIV testing. If your doctor or counselor thinks you should be tested, find out why and discuss the issue thoroughly. Remember, testing cannot hurt you or anyone else. You cannot get HIV from the test. If you are concerned about confidentiality, discuss it with your counselor and don't be shy. Ask all the questions you need to have answered. Health care providers work with many people who have questions, and they really want to help you.

AMBER: I'm very, extra safe. I didn't have sex with my fiancé until we were both tested for AIDS. We always use condoms, always have safe sex.
AUDREY: Lock yourself up in the room if you are manic (joke). Practice safe sex.
MARCUS: Safe sex: always use a condom. You should practice it.
SHARON: Use protection and don't get involved with a bunch of men. Make sure if you lie down with somebody that you love them and they love you.
LAURIE: No sex is good sex while you are recovering.

Additional HIV/AIDS resources:
www.cdc.gov/hiv/pubs/brochure.htm
www.cdc.gov/hiv/
www.fda.gov/oashi/aids/hiv.html
www.aegis.com
Living with HIV: A Patient's Guide, *Mark Cichok, 2009*
100 Questions and Answers About HIV and AIDS, *Joel E. Gallant, 2007*
The First Year. HIV: An Essential Guide for the Newly Diagnosed, *Brett Grodeck,*
2007

13 UNDER THE MICROSCOPE

After they get home from the hospital, most people say, their families and friends watch them very carefully to make sure that none of the old problems returns. Sometimes family members seem to be reminding them to take their medication several times a day. Attention like this can make you feel very uncomfortable. But remember, these are the same moms, dads, brothers, sisters, aunts, uncles, cousins, grandparents, and friends who walked through the halls of the psychiatric hospital to visit you. They will become more comfortable as you continue to recover—and so will you.

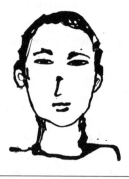

GARY

GARY: A lot of this is going to be distorted because it's not on my mind like it once was, but three years ago this would have been fresh on my memory. I think I had a pretty stressful year prior to the illness, but as I was living that year I didn't think so. Five years ago I graduated from high school. Immediately after that I got my driver's license and started working. Work was very stressful. I would work between 3 p.m. and midnight. Sometimes, there were days I worked eleven or twelve hours straight. Even though I was a pretty good student in high school, I was not prepared for college. I devoted less time to college than to work, so I didn't do so well. The first semester I ended up with a D, a C–, a C+, and a B–. This was different from the grades I had in high school, but it makes sense since I was spending less time on college than I had on high school. My second semester I took fourteen credits with the same crazy work schedule. My job was stressful, dealing with customers and the various procedures involved. It was spring four years ago when I failed two tests for one class, something I had never done before. I met with the professor and he gave me the opportunity to take it as an incomplete. I explained that to my father. He was kind of shocked, but he told me not to tell my mother. So all that summer it was on the tip of my mind—not that my mother would have been mad at me for failing a class. After my first two semesters I was placed on academic probation. That was very stressful. The threat at the time was that they would dismiss me from school. When I was nineteen years old I thought that was the end of the world, not working or going to school. But that was a nineteen-year-old reality.

Before I got sick I found myself studying more and more. I wasn't aware there was a problem. In October I was studying for midterms. I look back now and it's hard for me to believe what happened. I was admitted to the hospital on Thursday. On Sunday night prior to that I'd had trouble sleeping and had racing thoughts. I didn't think anything was wrong at the time. I just remember being really happy lying in bed that night. My breathing and heart rate started getting faster. I tried calming myself by pacing myself to my father's snoring in the next room. The next day when I came back from school I had to drive my brother somewhere. He told me I was driving fast and I stopped the car fast. I was listening to the radio, and I remember feeling very soothed by it. The song playing was "Up on the Roof." I was blasting it. That night again I had racing thoughts. That Tuesday I went to meet with the academic advisor. I was talking to her and I was saying outlandish stuff. I remember saying to her stuff that was very embarrassing for her. She replied, "Are you on drugs?" I said, "No." I remember sitting in her office. There was a bee in the window and I remember her being scared of the bee. I was thinking it was the same bee that had stung me several days before. Later, in class, I handed in a paper that reflected all my delusions. I remember writing something that was very metaphorical for one of my classes. I thought it made sense, but my mother thought I was very angry and it didn't make a lot of sense. I was sitting with friends who were taking a class with me, and I remember thinking that I was actually able to read their minds. I thought they were able to read my mind as well. They thought I was kidding around. As I left school that day I couldn't find my car. Finally I found it and returned home. I went to play the lottery, ten dollars' worth of the same numbers. I was picking the numbers out for one hour, and my father thought something was wrong. Then I really thought I was going to win. I remember taking a picture of [the ticket] to use as a press release for the newspapers. This was the third day into the episode, when my parents realized something was wrong. I thought I was making sense, but obviously I wasn't: I said, "See all the posters in my room, they all form a whole, and they are all interconnected." My parents called my brothers. I remember looking at my brother's face and it looked like his face was changing on me, turning into a monster. My brother started crying because he knew something was wrong. I remember myself going to the bathroom while they were all talking. I felt nauseated, but it was like hangover nausea. My stomach was tense for a half hour. My father was afraid something was going to happen and he slept in the bed with me. When they presented the idea of going to a psychiatrist, I didn't object. Deep inside I knew something was wrong. That morning the clocks were wrong. I thought my parents had changed the clocks for some reason. This was the third day that I didn't get any sleep.

I remember waiting in the walk-in clinic, all the patients sitting next to me. I thought it was some kind of game, that they were all actors and I was supposed to guess what role they were supposed to play. I remember looking at the clock in the waiting room and it was upside down. That was pretty scary. The person who admitted me asked if I would like to be admitted and I said yes. Once they brought me to Low III, I remember thinking that all of this was some type of show. I had never been in a psych hospital before, so I think it seemed to make all of my delusions more real. I had never been exposed to patients with these kinds of symptoms before. When I first was on the Low I was paranoid about my watch. I was so upset, they put me in the quiet room. So then I was alone in the quiet room with my watch. I remember looking at my watch and thinking that it had some sort of special power. I'm just telling you about the first week. That's nothing. I remember waking up in the quiet room and think-ing that one of the staff had had sex with me. I was very scared. For a week I actually believed that I had some fatal venereal disease. In the hospital I was depressed that I couldn't see my new nephew grow up. I would cry.

At home I was treated differently, in good ways and bad. It seemed like I had reverted. Here I was, a nineteen-year-old and being somewhat independent, and now my whole family was taking care of me like I was a child. I really didn't think about it much at the time because I just wanted to get well. I appreciated their help, my parents making sure I got my medication and my father driving me to the day hospital. I kind of liked the support because I was just so exhausted from the illness and from the side effects of the medication. I really needed that helping hand.

There was an expectation that I was supposed to get better quicker than I had; that's what my parents learned from attending workshops. I remember nine months into day hospital, the psychiatrist running into me saying, "So, when are you going back to school?" My father wanted me to go back to work four months after I was discharged, but my confi-dence was low and I had all these side effects. I also had to learn to have conversations again because I was out of practice due to the 130-day-long hospitalization, the illness, and the side effects from the medication.

JOSEPH: When I was in the hospital, my family was beyond supporting. They did not miss a visit. Besides my immediate family, friends, aunts, and uncles all showed me great support. My mom would come and sneak in home-cooked meals. Afterward, my parents were very worried; they would watch me, be a little more careful about what they said to me, how they acted around me. Basically, I went back to being a baby for a while. They wanted to know everything that happened. For example, when my grandfather passed away, naturally I cried. My grandmother kept coming up to me asking if I was going to be all right. She was worried I was going to break down. I responded by telling her she had nothing to worry about, that I was just sad. Inside I knew they were just looking out for my best interests. So I didn't take it personally.

SHARON: My parents were very understanding. My mother stood by me to the end. My mother just cared more; she gave me more love, more attention.

LUCINDA: I just felt that to my face my family didn't treat me differently. Probably behind my back they did talk about it. I feel that they did see me differently. They kept reminding me of my illness, which did not help me when I was discharged from the hospital. I would have preferred my family not to even mention the illness to me.

MIKE: I had a very understanding family. The one thing that would kind of get to me was the worry. I knew that they would worry a lot. I didn't want to see them worrying. I knew I was okay.

BUDDY: The last few years I was trying different kinds of help, like therapists and homeopathic medicine. My grandma always thought I was on drugs, smoking marijuana. She didn't know anything about schizophrenia. My mother, on the other hand, knew I had a problem, so she could understand what the staff was telling her. So she was happy I was finally being treated properly. My friends didn't know, so they didn't treat me any differently. Maybe one or two stopped coming around for a while. As soon as I started getting better, things were good.

GENEVIE: I don't think my family understood me at all. I was a burden. I was difficult. They couldn't understand how come all of a sudden I'm saying people are following me or my mother is trying to poison me. After I got out of the hospital they knew. I talked to them more easily. I have a better relationship with my family. They worry about me. My mother is always telling me to take my medication. After I leave for my apartment, she always yells after me, "Do you have your medication?" It's funny, one night she was taking her insulin and I was taking my medication and she said, "Everybody in the family is taking medication."

LAURIE: My family is doing really great. They know a lot about what I did before I got sick and they accept it. They don't bad-mouth me or hit me. They are just trying to cope with what I am going through. They used to get very mad at me when I used to do things. My mom and dad would hit me. I was always going out, not doing my chores, not listening to them. When I came home from the hospital my parents let me have my space.

SAMANTHA: My family still supports me and cares about me. I could go to my parents for just about anything. My parents watched me go down the drain slowly. They did not wish to have me live at home. They give me very little money. My dad has been struggling with an illness and he is not quite himself either. I just felt as though my mom had to focus most of her attention on him. Obviously they do treat me differently, but they want to help.

BETH: In the beginning when I first started taking the medication and getting better, my parents wouldn't let me drive. But after that, when they saw I was myself, they backed off and just let me be.

RICHIE: My family treated me normal. They didn't treat me like I was an outcast. If I feel apathetic, my father always tells me to fight it, to get a job. He treats me normal. He should, because I think if you treat somebody like they are sick, you baby them, you give them a crutch in life.

ZELDA: When you first get out of the hospital you are going to be a little child again. There are new rules. Your parents are very worried about you. They will ask you twice a day if you are going to take your medicine even if it's three in the afternoon and you're not supposed to take it until night. "Are you going to take your medicine?" They're just very overprotective.

PATRICK: They would watch me all the time. At first it was a little disturbing, because at first you can't handle it. You don't like to hear things like that, but you have to accept it.

MARCUS: When I first went home, my mom and dad used to stay in the room with me. They would watch me all the time to see if I was okay. It was tough for them to keep me on track. They would tell me there was nothing on the TV or radio, like cameras and stuff, people watching me; that there was nothing going on outside. It was scary, like I was a baby again. I was twenty-four years old and they were watching every move I made. It wasn't real comfortable in the beginning. I told them they could go to sleep, but every time I woke up they were there. They didn't get much sleep.

SMOKEY: My family didn't want me to go anywhere by myself. They thought I was going to drink beer and liquor and smoke weed. They were watching me carefully. Still, when I go somewhere and I come back, they check my breath and my hands. They make sure I take my medicine every night.

THOMAS: It bothers me a little bit when my mother reminds me to take my medicine because it makes me feel like a little kid.

BEN: I fought with my family because of me, not because of them. They were just trying to help. I was very stubborn about my views, which were all wrong. But my family was helpful. It bothered me that they watched me so carefully. I thought they didn't trust me. They asked if I took my medication. To me they were overly concerned, but the things they were worried about were totally appropriate. They were supposed to be worrying, but I didn't like it.

VAN: Actually, my family was really good about it. They were so glad to see me home. They didn't really treat me any special way. They still showed that they cared. They made sure I would continue with therapy and come to the hospital.

AMBER: When I first got sick my mother and father visited me at the hospital almost every morning. That helped a lot because I needed support from my family. My sisters visited me, and I found that very comforting because it made me feel I wasn't alone. My parents have been supportive of me trying to find a job and they haven't been putting any pressure on me. They told me to take my time.

BUCK: My family didn't know what to do when I got sick. They didn't know I was sick. I was just isolated from everybody. Sometimes it seems like my mom is putting pressure on me to go to the program, take my medication, stop hanging out. She doesn't want me to stay home. She doesn't want me to have any friends. Maybe she thinks my friends will do drugs and have me doing drugs and I'll end up back in the hospital.

ABBY: I don't want my mother worried about me. My mother will ask me, "Did you take your medication?" She notices when I talk about things like music and parties. Then she says, "You're doing good." My family jokes around sometimes.

JEFF: It's definitely an adjustment when you get home from the hospital. It's a lot of getting used to doing stuff again. My family saved the Christmas tree for when I got back so it felt like Christmas.

ALEXIS: My friends seemed understanding. They called me in the hospital, visited me, and they were my friends after the hospital. My mother wasn't so understanding and accepting of my being in the hospital. She would visit me every day, though. She would say things like, "They let you out of the hospital too soon, nut job." Then if I was spending money, she thought I was sick again. When I would go into the store she would think I was going to steal again. Even when I was well my mother would say derogatory things like "mental case." She would fly these words by like they were nothing. She would rather I had AIDS, cancer, anything but a mental illness.

She would say, "Why me, two nut jobs, you and your father." What really got me to go for therapy with her was her screaming "My daughter had a nervous breakdown" right in a doctor's office. And she told my friend. That was a violation of my privacy. In the beginning I would yell back and slam the door. I wouldn't deal with it calmly. So I went back to therapy. The therapy made me a better communicator, not only with my mom but with everybody. It helped my mom even though she didn't want to go in the beginning. It helped her cope with the illness and understand about the illness. It also made our relationship much better.

AUDREY: My family still babies me and tries to keep me in their nest. As an art student I'm not unusual. In high school it is harder, but it gets better. You may feel that you are under a microscope, but you would be surprised that there are people out there who are accepting of it.

This is Zelda's story. She wanted to explain in detail all the experiences she remembered. For most of us, reading Zelda's story was comforting. It reminded us that we shared many of the same thoughts, feelings, and behaviors, and that we really are not alone in this.

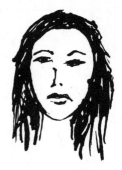

ZELDA

ZELDA: It doesn't ruffle my feathers too much to write about all that happened through the few days leading up to and during my six-week breakdown at the hospital. I think now I have a pretty good understanding of myself and my role in what I have been through and where I'm going.

They say Zelda wasn't Zelda for a few days until my parents came and picked me up from the University of Rochester. I know I hadn't slept more than a couple of hours in three days because I had a lot of schoolwork to do. I also wasn't eating too much—I was trying to become vegetarian, and did not have the taste for dining hall food. Plus, I had unresolved issues with one of my roommates, which was caused by poor choices that I had made. I guess the pressure was getting to me, but I didn't realize that there was a huge problem on the rise. I knew something wasn't right. My thoughts were starting to run circles around each other and I was experiencing some paranoia. I don't know who called them, but one of my friends called my parents, who then insisted that they come and get me right pronto.

171

The long eight-hour ride was horrible. When we stopped at a motel in Rochester, I did not sleep at all. The whole night I thought my father was speaking to me—or to someone, maybe my mom, maybe himself—through his snores. Every breath, in and out, was a phrase. In the car ride home my parents had a book on tape that seemed to dictate to me: my life and my mistakes or tiny secrets. In a coffee shop that we stopped at to get a bite to eat, I believed that the two older men next to us were talking about me, under their breath. As we got up to leave I yelled at them, "Have a good day." Everything was wrong.

When we got home, I mostly stayed in my bed. I grabbed pants off the messy floor that I actually hadn't seen in years (how they got there, I'm not sure) and though they should have been too small for my body, they slipped off me. Maybe because, having not eaten in days, I was thinner—my little potbelly shrinking rapidly. My parents gave me a sleeping pill to induce the much-needed rest, and they tried to offer me food. But as I was lying in my bed, the smell of Chinese food on my night table was rotting in my nose like vomit. Food needs to smell good to entice us to eat. Well, I wanted no part of it. I "realized" so much about the need for this and that, why this is this way and that is that way, blah blah blah. Like a bad trip, my thoughts were overloaded, overwhelming, and overanalytical. And that was just when I was alone. But then someone would walk in (to check on me, to offer me something, to tell me we had to go see the doctor), and my confusion would soar. During that time in my bedroom I wrote in my spiral book from school. I wrote all over it in phrases and fragments and conclusions. I drew circles, outlining how all the thoughts fit together and formed a cycle. My thoughts were wild and out of hand.

When my parents took me to the psychiatrist, she gave the direction: ZUCKER HILLSIDE HOSPITAL.

It was late at night and it was fairly dark in the hallway when the lady wearing a nurse's outfit walked me into my room. She asked me all kinds of questions, with her clipboard in hand. I remember lying to some of her questions just for the hell of it—it didn't matter to me; I didn't even know what the truth was anymore. And I don't know why I remember this, but she took her shoe off in the middle of the interview. She must have had a long day. She left for a minute or thirty minutes and came back with some "medicine," which looked to me like a medicine cup filled with orange juice, and a large cup of o.j. to wash it down with. One flew over the cuckoo's nest. I thought they were conning me as to what I needed to "get better."

I'm not sure if I slept at all that night, but I do remember being startled by the voices in the hallway the next day. I hadn't realized the night before when I was brought through quiet halls that there were many other people sharing the space. What was this place? I sort of believed that the voices out there were a fake scene and it was all planted for my benefit. A logical question like, "Why in the world would it be planted for me?" never entered my scattered mind. When it comes to paranoia, nothing is logical.

My parents came that day with a duffel bag of clothes and a little plastic "Bloomies" toilet kit. Had I packed my own bag in the condition I was in, it might have held the same contents; but on a regular day, I never would have chosen these clothes. I didn't make a stink about it. (No offense to my parents, or their fashion sense. My point is to show that any ounce of my style, inside and out, was sucked dry, so that I didn't care what I looked like—or what I felt like.) They also gave me a legal pad and a pen, which seemed pretty random, but I subsequently made use of it. One night, it may have been that night, I wrote in fierce anger, covering every page—right up to the cardboard backing. Those poems would be very interesting to read now. Unfortunately, shortly after I had filled the pad, I was in the day room drawing on the back cover. Someone asked me what I was holding. I said, "NOTHING!" and threw the whole thing in the garbage. It's too bad. But at that point nothing mattered—not my words, my looks, my *health*, or my confidence, which was zero.

Getting me out of my room at all during my hospital daze was not an easy job for the workers of Zucker Hillside Hospital, but the first few days may have been the most trying. The first time I braved the walk down the hall for a meal, which was chicken something, I couldn't even bring myself to take a tray. (In the beginning of your stay in the hospital, a wheeled table is brought into the common room—a.k.a. the day room—and someone serves the meals before mysteriously disappearing. When you gain status—a crazy privilege title—you make the trek out into another area of the hospital: the cafeteria.) Eating was hard for me at first, but I think the scariest thing about going to meals was the necessary eye contact with others, the pure fear of being around anyone—feeling like an art exhibit to be gawked at and analyzed.

Eating and drinking caused another undesired endeavor. The trips to the public, dormlike bathrooms were torturous for me. The first time I went into one, a lady, maybe in her mid-thirties, looked at me and let out a low-volume, low-emotion "Hi," meaning: "Hi, you're the new girl? We're all in this together. Grin and bear it." Her hair was up in a sloppy, curly ponytail; her face was lacking makeup and happiness. I vocalized nothing in return, but my face said to her, "Please just ignore me. I'm only in here because I couldn't hold it in anymore. My first choice would be to pee all over the floor in my room, but then I would have to associate with that man with the mop." Maybe she didn't hear all that with my expression. Probably she just quickly got the notion that I was as hopeless as she looked.

After what seemed to be a few days (it would be interesting to check the files and find out how long it really was) I was transferred to Low III, another ward in the hospital. Here I began eating more substantially. The problem was that I couldn't stand the idea of food, or the taste of it in my mouth. An analogy that I will draw will be understood by anyone who has ever had too much alcohol. It's been a party night and you've been drinking for hours and hours, and by now you are in the bathroom, by the bowl, in between heaves. Your head is spinning and nausea is your best friend. Now I'm standing by you with a bottle of vodka, telling you that you have to chug. Can you feel the comparison? Even if you've never been so sloppy drunk, maybe you can just imagine this. The situations are different in one significant aspect, however. The distinction is that vodka may have sent you to your deathbed, but food is necessary to sustain life. And the people at Zucker Hillside were not going to let me die. When I realized this, I knew I had to eat something, and this was the first turning point of my experience. The understanding was that there was no self-destruction in this damn hospital.

Even the fact that my parents and my brother came every day to visit didn't matter. Although I liked seeing them, I almost wanted them to stop coming because their support clashed with my insanity; I wanted to be left alone with my crazy mind and unnourished body. Now, of course, I know that their company was very essential to my feat of gaining control and sparked a reason to get back on my feet and *live*.

As it sounds, it was incredibly (if that's even a strong enough word) negative in every aspect. I was so paranoid, and at the same time depressed. I felt that everyone in the hallway was talking about me but was too down on myself to care. I felt everything was fraud. People would come into the room and, as if on cue, someone would check my "vitals." Staff people would roll in a device that checked my blood pressure. They listened with their stethoscopes and touched my skin with their hands to hold it on the inside of my elbow. And they took my pulse. But the thing that made me assume that the whole charade was fake was the thermometer. They put this plastic on a rod, put it in my mouth, and pressed a button. The mechanical arrow bleeped around in a circle. Sanitation was the last thing on my mind, and I thought it was an obvious prop. Why did they need to be checking all this anyway? They may have explained that it was to monitor my body for side effects of the medicine they put me on, but even if they had tried to, my mind would have rejected the facts and concocted some other explanation. What made it more surreal was the fact that while I was out in the day room, they only took "vitals" from a select few.

There were patients and there were workers planted in this nightmare. And those times I came out of my room to walk down that terrible hallway, having to make humanoid contact, it was totally unclear to me who the workers—social workers, doctors, interns—were. In a glass cabinet there were Polaroid pictures with names under them of our "staff friends." Some of these faces were familiar and some weren't. From this I deducted that the display was another ploy, like so many things, to fool me and some other insanos. So I made assumptions with the rest of the cast and pinpointed those working and those living in these rooms with light blue blankets on the beds.

Walking down the hall, petrified as a mouse, I wanted to float myself into invisibility. But they really wanted me to come out from my foxhole. I can swear that one time they came and got me from my room, put me in a big old dentist's chair, and wheeled me into the day room. I can kind of remember my parents being there. Maybe I refused to leave my room for so long, they had to devise a plan to integrate me as an upstanding member of the unit. (If this was the reason I was wheeled and placed out there, I just have to laugh.) I'm not really so sure why that happened. As so many unexplained scraps go, it still gets filed under the paranoid delusions. Perhaps it was just a dream.

Another source of confusion rang in the halls and left different impressions on me as time went on. The first time I heard the phone ring outside my room, I thought it was God calling and I let someone else answer. (I had no idea what to say to him.) After a few different times, I realized that there was a real phone in the hallway and it wasn't some spiritual passageway. But at this point, I thought that people in the other hall were calling in an attempt to get me out of my room and see what I was all about. I was in no condition to meet people or be social, so I just let it ring. One time, however, I did peep out and answer it, to find that they weren't looking for me at all. And even though the phone wasn't for me (maybe it was for Sharon, or Tony, I don't remember), somehow the call was still only for my benefit—just to see what I would say. The phone calls were still just a prop on this bizarre set. For a while this Spanish woman (I can remember her looks very distinctly, as I can with certain people in this ordeal) would stay on the phone for what seemed an hour, just repeating "Si, Billy, Si, Billy," in her nasal voice. I can't figure out what this guy Billy kept asking, day after day, but didn't he get the point? I don't know if I thought that she was actually talking to someone. My conviction at the time may have been that this "phone conversation" was her creative release. Another lady walked around with a jug of iced tea. Another girl had a tiny tape player, which always played the song "Zombie" by the Cranberries. Anyway, everybody had something. So the "Si, Billy" lady may have just had the telephone. Toward the end of my episode, I used the phone myself to call Rochester to see how things were up there and sort of let them know I was alive. This was a step on my healing ladder. I was extremely shaky on the line, but it went over fine, and I have since talked to my old roommates to find that things are not left untied.

There is a little kindling of thought in the back of my mind that I could have survived my few days of emotional and mental anarchy in Rochester without being rushed home and put away. Some part of me wonders what would have happened if a good friend sat with me until I was "me" again. Just like those few times I got high and bugged out, when I just needed a hand to hold, so to speak, until I realized how backward I was thinking. Then I would not have spent six weeks in the hospital. And I wouldn't have "schizophrenia," and I wouldn't be on a leash (clozapine) that makes decisions for me—no drinking (a former habit of mine), and when to go to sleep so that I have enough time to be jelly on my medication. However, first of all, I believe that all things happen for a reason. And second, I think I'm in a good place now and I might not be so good if I'd been permitted to go wild. While some experts may call it denial, there's that little piece of me that wonders. A very little piece.

I know that during this breakdown I was stripped of all my personality and soul. In the emergency room, before I even got to Zucker Hillside, I gave my mom my necklaces (I wore three, each with significant meaning). And two major things were robbed from me: music and dance. Any music that played was analyzed, and the paranoia that turned everything to negativity, self-consciousness, and indecency roared to every song. Of course, I also couldn't dance. I believe one time, when I was in my room alone, I tried to bust a move but stopped after a fast unsuccessful swivel. I felt someone watching and judging and it just wouldn't work. Now, I don't care who's watching; if I get the urge to dance I'll have no trouble. And that's the way it should be. Why should I care what people are thinking if I'm just trying to get down? I can remember when music started to come back to me. It may have been after about a month, a month and a half. I was walking alone outside, on my way back from the Activities Therapy building, when I started singing (to myself), "If I ran away, I'd never have the strength to go very far, how will they hear the beating of my heart. . . ." Madonna! Of all artists, of all my favorite music before I was sick, why was it Madonna? Who knows? Some would try to analyze. But it was a pretty good feeling to be able to sing again and not think twice.

My body showed the picture of mental malfunction. I lost about ten, fifteen pounds. Pimples popped out all over my back and some on my face. My lips were scabbed and frowns tore down my dispirited eyes. I had a hacking cough. One night, shortly after I was put on medication, I woke up to puke in my garbage can. As I walked down the dark, vacant hallway to get rid of the bag of vomit, the hall guards asked where I was going. I gave no reply. I guess this new chemical in my body generated the throw up. One day while I was in my room (alone) I had a seizure. What an amazing thing it was. It just came on out of nowhere. I can remember trying to hold onto the bed as I lost all control of my body and was jerked violently, as if a big, invisible giant shook the shit out of me. It's not as though I thought there was someone there I couldn't see. I sort of knew it was from the medicine, or something they had done to me (maybe the CAT scan or the EKG). What a scary experience, though, added to the list of uncontrollable terrors. And I really believe that all that I was thinking, all my perceptions, were as hard to restrain as a seizure. They came on like gangbusters. One needs incredible strength to hold themselves still when the chemical and electrical parts of the body dysfunction enough to tremble. But some shakes are powerful enough that all the strength in the world can't reject them. This analogy may sound like a cop-out. I do say now that you must not back down to the challenge of control when it comes to your body (and mind).

My advice to others experiencing a "psychotic episode" would be subjective. By this I mean, it would depend on the person and their experience. My experience was predominantly ruled by paranoia, delusions, and extremely low self-confidence. But those are just descriptive words to categorize thoughts or feelings. Each person is going through her or his own thing. It is hard to determine what advice would be helpful for anyone, let alone for myself at that time.

I can drop some suggestions to those who love the ill. I don't remember anyone grabbing me and saying, "*Snap out of it, girl!*" It might have been okay to play it down a bit, even laugh a little at me. Even though the situation was serious, it might have been helpful if people didn't take me and my wacky behavior so heavily. I do remember my brother smiling (with heart behind his eyes) and saying something like, "Seriously, Zelda, what's up?" I think we may have even shared a laugh. This is the type of thing that helped my soul, because he had faith that somewhere inside my sad-looking body I was still there, and he knew he could bring me out with a true smile. I can say that support, whether it's many visits or unfailing faith, and one thing like homemade oatmeal raisin cookies, will definitely benefit that crazy person. My parents stood by me very close

177

and I can say now, in retrospect, that their presence was very important. (Can't we say so many things in retrospect?)

The healing process is a very long one, and we human beings tend to be short-attention-spanned impatients (my word). It will take some work to regain yourself after a psychotic fit, but mostly it just takes time. I remember while I was in Zucker Hillside, workers and my parents were telling me it was going to take time. I didn't even know what it was, but the idea was planted, and, man, does it take time. While your mind is playing games with you and all of your energy is spent negatively, you are tearing down walls of learning you've built over the years. When you first get out of the hospital you will probably feel like a helpless child again. And, in a sense, you pretty much are. They say that this disease first appears in eighteen- to twenty-two-year-olds. These can be big party years for some people. You might have been used to hanging out with your friends, downing a few or smoking a few, or whatever your pleasure was, and staying out late having fun (without many restrictions). All of a sudden you are caged in for weeks in a crazy place. Then you're out and, of course, you don't just snap into who you were before you got sick. Now your parents are making rules you haven't had since you were twelve, curfews and all. And maybe your friends are treating you differently and acting different. (Hey, they did a lot of changing too while you were away.) This is in addition to the fact that your brain is in neutral, trying to heal its broken self. And this takes: time.

Right after people have a heart attack, they are ordered to give attention to their health, and if they want to live they will listen. Their whole way of living is usually changed. All of a sudden they have to eat differently. All of the unhealthy foods (which may have been their favorites) are forbidden. Anything that could be a stressor is eliminated to a point that their hearts are no longer at risk. Now, I suppose there is a difference in the end result of a heart attack: death. For a psychotic episode it's a bad time in a mental hospital (and perhaps a chance of permanent insanity). But the theme is identical. It is a shocking shake-up that has to be paid attention to and nursed to recovery. The time after my episode was pretty rough. In the very beginning I had to go to day hospital, which I can remember comparing to Purgatory. There were all these programs to boost self-esteem and social skills and such. I still wasn't myself yet but was no longer paranoid by then (as I recall). Quite a step from my hospitalized self; still, I was not at all what I wanted to be. I wanted to be with my friends. On the weekends I couldn't party or stay out late. After a month of day hospital, there was group therapy and medicine to take and side effects to handle. I was nowhere near my old self (or myself now). But eventually, after proving myself saner, I was able to have a lower dose on my meds and change the frequency of my group therapy meetings to every other week, then not at all. (I still see my social worker once a month.) And by some great miracle, the blood they take from me to test my white blood cell count is only taken every other week now.

I must say that an enormous help to my psyche was and is my private therapist, whom I used to see every week and now I go to every other week. I am very lucky to have been able to see her; I've learned so much from those visits, it's amazing. It's different for everyone, and for some, seeing a shrink is not their ball game, but if it is possible to try I would definitely recommend it. Before I got sick I wasn't too keen on the idea for reasons of self-absorption (basically sitting around talking about yourself for an hour), financial reasons, and privacy reasons (who should know the deep thoughts I have but me?). Well, it's helped me, for whatever reasons, so I am very grateful. It is a long process indeed, but you need two things and you've got good chances. Number one is patience. (Remember, if there's one thing in this world we can count on, it's that time will keep passing.) Number two is a strong will to want to get better and achieve it. To do this you will need to make sacrifices, which in the long run will be to your benefit.

There's a fine line we all walk with insanity. When I meet people now (post-psychotic bout), at some point I have to explain that I was in a mental hospital for some time. I am categorized as "schizophrenic" and I'm on antipsychotic drugs. People do not believe that I was ever psychotic, mainly because I am not psychotic now. And, you see, I believe that we are all insane—what is a straight mind? It's creativity and imagination that our minds use, or logic or deduction or protection or judgment. It's every rationale that we make for things and every game we play. It's our own personalities and it's all subjective. The question is whether these traits, these inner workings of the mind, cause us to hurt ourselves or other people. Can we exist and work things out? When we can't, there is a problem. I heard every conversation in the hallway, every interpersonal connection in some way pecking at my being. And I could not stop this. I lost control.

And this is dangerous insanity.

Now I don't have that problem. The voices in a hallway are just that—people who are having their own conversations. And even if they are talking about me, for any reason, I don't care. I'll even laugh with them (or at them). This world is a crazy place, but I have to do the best that I can. I have too much to give to waste time being an invalid. And I have one more thing to say about this. One of the myriads of questions I am asked monthly to see if I am sane (or to keep tabs on my "disease") is: "Do you think you are special in any way?" Maybe if I were insanely paranoid, this question would screw with my head. Being of sound mind and body, though, I laugh and answer yes—everyone is special. Sorry if it sounds like a line straight out of *Harold and Maude*, but we all have something special that makes us who we are—different people. We shouldn't be cardboard cutouts. If my tone sounds a bit defensive here, maybe it's because I am. I guess there are a few things to be defensive about when it comes to my personality and my mental illness.

I write this story as a means of putting my experience in words so that I can learn more *from* it, and so that others can maybe understand it from my point of view. But perhaps you had similar experiences and now see that you are not alone. All I can say is that although we may never fully understand this brain disease, we can live with it and have productive lives. We just need ways of expressing ourselves. For me, words do the trick.

15 WHO AM I NOW?

This is everyone's favorite chapter, because here we tell you what is happening in our lives now. Some of us are doing very well. Others have had a tougher time getting or staying on the road to recovery. This may be because we didn't take our medication or had a harder time finding the right one, or it might be because we used drugs or alcohol. But for all of us this chapter is a testimony to the fact that life goes on and there is hope for a future.

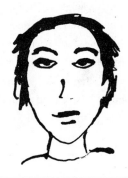

JOSEPH

JOSEPH: I'm not ashamed of my illness. Everybody has problems in life. Some people seek help and others don't. In my case, I was eighteen when I discovered my illness. I had a lot of problems at home. My father left. There wasn't a lot of income, and it put a lot of pressure on my shoulders.

Then out of nowhere, symptoms started creeping up on me. I believed that I was being followed by the FBI. My phones were being tapped, video cameras were set up in my house, and I couldn't even trust my friends or my family. When my mom was on the phone I really believed that she was talking about me to the FBI. When this happened, at first I thought maybe I was just being paranoid, but as the days went on and the symptoms didn't go away I realized that I needed help. That is when I checked myself into the hospital. But at first I thought the hospital was a detention center for the FBI. And even when I first came in, things didn't get any better; they actually got worse. I was thrown into a new environment that I had never been in before, which was very scary. At that point in time I started to become suicidal. I didn't think life was worth living. I thought that being dead was the right answer. So about two days after being in the hospital I made an attempt at my own life, which, thank God, did not succeed. From that point on it still didn't get any better, but at least I had back the will to live. The will to live came back partly through speaking with other patients. When I spoke with people at the time they told me way more frightening stories than I'd ever experienced. One man told me he was raped by a relative when he was eight years old and went on to tell me other unimaginable things. That was when I realized that my life wasn't too bad. From that point on I started to regain my consciousness. I started to become myself again, laugh again, enjoy my family's company; to actually enjoy life and have fun. Even when I left the hospital, there was still a lot of work to be done. I still needed continuous care. At first I tried to revolt and told myself, "I am fine now, everything is okay. I don't need a doctor. I don't need a therapist." It took me almost a year to realize that my illness was nothing to be ashamed of and, in some way, shape, or form, I had to cope and deal with it. Which I did, thanks to the doctors and therapists.

Now, four years later, I have turned my life completely around. I've learned to deal with my illness and go on with my everyday life. Not as a psychotic person who has problems and can't be in reality. I am just like everybody else, what society would consider a normal person. I am now attending college, getting good grades, holding a steady relationship with a very nice girl, and I look forward to completing my education, and, furthermore, becoming an accountant. I have daily structure now, something to live for.

ABBY: Now I'm up to the point where I've tried the shock treatment. I'm trying to get help because my emotions are being controlled and my thoughts are being controlled. Sometimes it even feels like my movements are being controlled. It bothers me that the symptoms bother me. I just want to get better.

ALEXANDRA: I'm doing much better since I've been out of the hospital for four years. I'm happy that I'm out, that I can get to places I want to go to. I'm not depressed anymore. I'm happy to go out, do what I have to do, take care of the house, and take care of my grandmother. And I'm happy that I can be there for my family.

ALEXIS: First I was diagnosed with schizoaffective disorder. Then two years later I was diagnosed with bipolar disorder. They gave me lithium for the first time, and it was working very well. With the lithium I was able to go back to college, taking a smaller workload at first and then working up to four classes, and then graduating college. I thought I would never do it, but I did. Out of college I immediately started to work as an assistant teacher for a year, and then I went to the board of education as a teacher. That job was a lot of stress. During the three months that I worked there I was aware of symptoms—not eating and not sleeping. I immediately brought myself into the emergency room and the doctor gave me sleeping pills. I realized my health was more important and I quit that job. I was devastated, but I went back to being an assistant teacher. I wasn't happy about it, but it was what I had to do. And then with therapy I gained back my confidence. I went back and got a new teaching job with a lot of stress, but I'm able to handle it—but only with the medicine. I'm definitely leading a wonderful life. I got engaged a month ago, and we are getting married this year.

AMBER: Right now I am looking for a job and I am trying to get on with my life. I haven't had any symptoms for two years. Life is great. I like hanging out with my family and friends. I try to take better care of myself, like I eat healthier now. After this incident I realized that the most important things in life are your friends and family, because they are the ones who supported me throughout this whole incident. I think things happen for a reason; at the time I was under a lot of stress, and I look back on it and think that maybe at the time I wasn't ready to be working at a job. I was very nervous at the workplace. My confidence was very low. Now I am very confident that I can perform well at a job. When I look back, I think maybe it wasn't such a bad thing that this happened to me. Maybe it happened for a reason.

AUDREY: Every year I go through severe depression in the fall. I have been hospitalized every fall since, but I find with each bout of depression I come out on the other end stronger and find that I have a great will to survive. I feel that my illness has enabled me to learn many things about myself. Also, I feel that it made me mature more quickly. If I had a choice to not have this illness I would decline. It is part of who I am, and for all the pain it's put me through, I have found it valuable in finding a greater depth in life. My accomplishments outweigh the setbacks my illness has caused me. I have confidence that I will have a successful and full life.

BEAUX: This illness changed me. It helped me to appreciate life and people around me. Everything came out positive. At my job I feel like I put in 110 percent. I try not to judge people. While I was in the hospital my relationship with my fiancée was on hold, but now we are together.

BEN: I'm still improving. It's a never-ending process. Every single day you learn. Every single day you improve. Right now I'm going to school. I'm going to college. Last summer I was a camp counselor. I also tried real estate for a short while. I worked in stores as a salesperson. They all turned out well. I left on my own for the next job. I made mistakes. Next year I'm going to be in charge of thirty people in my job. Basically, I'm getting my college degree and I'm looking forward to many things in the rest of my life. I think I'm going to do all of them. In the future, when I have a car, I hope to start dating. Life is for me to create now. I feel great. If you work hard, then trust me, it will work out.

BETH: Once you get used to taking the medication and you become stable, you pretty much live like everybody else. You have the potential to do whatever you want to do. I'm working as a physical therapist, which is what I wanted to do before I got sick. I'm dating somebody. I have my own apartment. I'm happy.

BUCK: My life is still rough. I'm not able to function as I did before I got sick. Before I could handle pressures of working or going to school, but now it's harder. Sometimes I feel hopeless, but I still have hope. I want to be able to get my GED and get a job. I have a little daughter. She brings me happiness. When I look at her it makes me want to do more, but with the illness sometimes it feels impossible. I still try to do the things I can. I still go to see her, play with her, let her know she has a daddy, and I'll

184

always be around. And that is what makes me look forward to having a normal life again.

BUDDY: Basically, I don't see myself as a person with schizophrenia right now. I leave that in the past. Right now I am just trying to live a normal, productive life. Hopefully it won't come back to haunt me if I keep coming to group, seeing my psychiatrist, and taking my medicine. After a year I'm working full-time, I'm back to writing, I'm looking forward to going back to college, and I have a girlfriend. I'm in a nice relationship.

GARY: I never thought I would be where I am right now. Actually, life has improved since I went into the hospital. I find myself being much more open to people and much more sympathetic as a result of all the therapy and what happened to me. I find myself being friendlier than I was prior to the illness. I'm working eighteen hours a week at my old job and I'm still in the same school. Now I'm an upper junior. I returned to college part-time and now I'm full-time. I've done the best I've ever done in school. I seem to be much happier because I get things off my chest better than I had been. I just started dating, a year and a half after my discharge date. I'm also in a club at school that involves what I want to do when I graduate. So, there is life after the illness.

GENEVIE: I see things more clearly now. I'm able to analyze things. I know the difference between what is real and what is not. I'm a little bit more open. Before I used to be afraid of people, but now I'm communicating more. I want to have friends. I don't know how to be with friends, how to deal with people. I think they will probably hurt me. I'm afraid of getting hurt. That's my next goal, to be able to have friends. When I was sick I thought I didn't have a future. I was pessimistic, and nothing good was going to come out of anything that I did. Now it's different; I have a goal. I'm going to school and I intend to get a job later on in life. It's good that I know a lot about my illness because I feel that if I'm getting sick again I can recognize the illness and go and get help. I'm glad I know about it. Here it's controlled, everybody is mentally ill. I have people to talk to, people who are dealing with the same thing I was dealing with. And it seems everybody wants to go forward with their lives. Everybody has a goal they want to accomplish.

ILAN: It's been five years now since my last breakdown. Three years ago I got my own apartment. I have returned to college, which is something I wanted to do. I was in a community college, but I graduated and I'm now pursuing a bachelor's degree at a four-year college in elementary education and sociology. I plan on a master's in education and a master's in social work. I don't believe college is for everyone, but it was something that was made important to me when I was younger. I plan to continue till I finish my goals, whether they change or not. It's good, for the most part, but as I go along I have to remember that new problems will come up along with the old ones. And I may have to learn new coping skills. It helps to look back and see all the other problems that I put in the drawer and closed.

My first semester back at my community college, I took a social work course and schizophrenia came up. There were things that were said that I was offended by. One girl said that her father laughs if someone is schizophrenic, and that hurt me. But I learned to ignore it or listen without letting the offense bother me. After a while it became easy to ignore stupidity, as we all have to ignore a lot of it. As to who I am now, I'm a lot better than I was before I broke down the first time. The doctors are worried about us, if we are going to fail. I have some worries, but I know that even if it's not a high-paying job, I will be successful in what I am doing. I can sit within myself and be comfortable.

JACKIE: Over the past few years I've been experimenting with what to do to keep myself well. I stopped drinking alcohol and I've stayed well ever since. I try to keep a structured life, as far as a schedule during the week, so I have things to do. That keeps me focused rather than in a dreamy world.

JAMES: Now my life is pretty much back on track. I feel good. I'm working, getting set to go back to school. My family is much better; I'm getting along with them. I'm not going to lie—sometimes I don't take the medicine and I start getting certain symptoms, like the headaches. But I am able to do things I was doing. So it's not really a bad thing; I'm doing maybe even more than before I went into the hospital.

JEFF: I'm doing okay. I get along with the people at work. I've been there a year. I'm doing all right. I don't have too many problems. Day by day, I take it as it comes. I'm not worrying about stuff that doesn't happen anymore. I'm trying to have as much fun as I can. I'm planning to go to Grand Cayman for a scuba-diving trip this summer. I'm going to book it soon. I'll do some refresher dives before I go. All in all, life is pretty good. I can't complain.

LAURIE: I feel much safer. Hopefully I will have good memories that will last me for a long time. I plan to go to college, but I'm still depending on the hospital for security.

LINDA: I am a struggling artist who wants to get stronger in her fight for survival and acceptance of this medication. I struggle to have a normal life, a family, and a job. Right now I am a person who goes to a day program, who has a boyfriend, and who pretty well maintains herself in life. I am living in QSLP, an apartment program. I also go to political advocacy groups for mentally ill people and I go to meetings for my apartment program's newsletter. I am going to start to play on a softball team. I go to the movies with my boyfriend and my friends. I Rollerblade. You can have a normal, active daily routine type of living after you have come out of the hospital. There are plenty of people who are on medication but have a normal life.

LUCINDA: I am the same person. Just carry on taking the medication and working and living your life as if there is nothing wrong with you. Don't be thinking about it all the time. If you are hospitalized again, you are hospitalized again. I have had three or four miserable years that I would not like repeated. I will do all I can not to have that repeated. I think I have learned a lot and I think I can prevent a repeat of those horrible years. I was always a strong person, but this has made me a much stronger person. I just want to work and get on with my life.

MARCUS: Now I can look back and say I had a sickness. It was real bad in the beginning, but now I'm getting back to my old self. It's something I have to deal with. I'm hanging out with my friends now. I have a job and I have a girlfriend. You can date with the sickness. It's okay to get a good night's rest, get up fresh, and start a new day.

MEREDITH: I am trying to finish college and take care of myself at the same time. I am enjoying singing in my choir. I am deepening my relationship with family. I traveled this summer to Japan and Mexico and had a wonderful time in both places. I have friends from choir and friends who graduated from college who are supportive.

MIKE: Well, I am doing much better now. I am enjoying life. I'm trying to stay more positive and be more positive about what the future has for me. I've learned to appreciate life and I am grateful to be alive, because there were times I didn't want to be alive at all. I look forward to keeping on taking my medicine, taking care of myself, and getting back into college. Just enjoying life to the fullest.

PATRICK: I think I am doing well. The exercise is keeping my mind in good shape. I would like to lose a lot of weight. I like my job. I meet people there and talk to other people.

RICHIE: I think I am doing pretty good except for my weight. I am doing much better than I was before. In time all that goes away, the apathy. I feel I'm back to my original self. I am trying to get back into working out and to find a job that I really like and stick with it. I'm going to call VESID (see appendix 2 for more information on VESID) and see if I can get help from them, to see if they can put me into a program to eventually put me into a job.

ROMAN: I am hoping to get a job. I'm hoping to move out of the apartment program and live on my own. I feel good.

SAM: I am more confident than I have been in seven years. I know I am doing well in school. I was offered a job at school. People having confidence in me helps me have confidence in myself. I can still learn things quickly. I think I'm a hundred times more humble. The sickness made me humble and, maybe because of this, I have many more friends than before. I still have the individuality, but not the arrogance anymore.

Now I'm in school and doing A work in the field I love. I think there's no reason not to expect a normal life. I'm happy with it.

SAMANTHA: It's a struggle. I sometimes have to take ten minutes at a time. I try to keep myself involved, occupied. I try to communicate with my little girl as much as possible. I'm alive. I see the sun rise in the morning. I can walk, I can talk, and I can feed myself. I can say if something physically is hurting me. I'm trying to work into a more professional job situation. I have been employed as an assistant case manager for the past four years. I have obtained my real estate license. I love activities. I do Jazzercize a couple times a week. I square dance. I like to walk. I like to read. I'm going to be starting a new job I was highly recommended for. It should be a step up for me to grow into. As my daughter gets older, I hope to be able to be more honest with her about myself. We have a good relationship now. Normal for a mother and teenager.

SASHA: Now I don't clean my house as much. I have plans to go to school, to start a business career. I bought a car to visit friends and family. I live alone in my own apartment. I am independent. My son lives with his father, and I see him on a regular basis. I am seeing someone, more like a friend, though. I feel good. I am bored a lot, though, because I am not working, but I don't have the symptoms I used to have.

SHARON: It's hard for me to deal with because I don't like to be classified with an illness. I still don't like to be labeled. My life stopped. My dancing, my schooling were put on hold. It seems like I'm never going to get it back again.

SMOKEY: Things are going okay. I go to school; I go see my counselor twice a week. Once a week I see my drug counselor. Every morning they search me. I feel very good about myself. I hope to finish school and get a job. I have a girlfriend. She calls every day.

THOMAS: It's been four years. I feel like I have gotten a little bit better. Hopefully the medication will help me. I feel pretty good. I'm waiting to see if my new medication helps me feel better.

VAN: Well, I've since pursued my education, and I'm looking forward to a career in the field of respiratory therapy. I have remained sharp and intelligent when it comes to learning in school. I've also continued to work throughout going to school. I go out with friends on the weekends and still enjoy good movies. I'm not leading a very exciting life. I think I have come back to the place in my life where I was long before I became ill. I've returned to a clearer head and a healthier attitude.

VANESSA: My life is coming together slowly. After my mother's death I was feeling a little bit lost, but now I'm feeling a little bit better, better about myself. I moved into my mother's house. When I moved in all the walls came down, the ceiling came down. There was so much work to do. She kept a lot of papers. I had to go through the papers to find certain bills, the deed to the house. Once we found all those papers we got everything together. The house is in better shape. Slowly but surely we are getting it together. We are adding a few things Mom would like. We're painting, getting the bathroom fixed. We've even got the kids painting. They are enjoying themselves. My son is doing much better in school and my daughter is my wonder girl. She is just doing her own thing. She is reading well, doing math well. She reads a lot. She was an honor student this year. Everything is coming along nice. I'm feeling much better. I can talk about my feelings now. Talk about the things that I do every day. That's it.

ZELDA: I am just trying to do the best I can with what I've been given. I'm working two jobs. I finished my two-year degree and I'm going on to become a massage therapist. I'm on a constant search to find the beautiful aspects of life and to keep things in perspective. I have been able to travel and make friends and stay sane. I think good health leads to productivity. So I am conscious of my well-being and am eating healthier, doing yoga, and staying on top of my game.

190   *Note: Mark contributed to the book in many ways but did not provide his story.*

16 GETTING THE SOCIAL SERVICES YOU NEED

There are so many things to worry about when you are first hospitalized for schizophrenia. First people worry about whether they will get well. Then they worry about paying the bills for the hospital, the doctors, their medication, and living expenses. These are legitimate concerns.

Many people get financial assistance and health insurance benefits from government-sponsored programs, in particular, Social Security, Medicaid, and Medicare. Even if you do not currently require assistance, it is important to know if you qualify for it and when it makes sense to apply. Here is some very basic information about social services. If you need to know more, talk to the person you work with in treatment or use the phone numbers and Web sites that are listed in this chapter and in the appendices.

SSI AND SSD—SUPPLEMENTAL SECURITY INCOME AND SOCIAL SECURITY DISABILITY INSURANCE

The U.S. government provides both SSI and SSD for people who cannot work because they are ill. The major difference between them is that SSI is for people who were not working when they first became ill, and SSD is for people who were working. For SSI, benefits begin on the first full month after you file, if your application is approved; for SSD there is a five-month waiting period from the time your disability began to the time you receive benefits. For both SSI and SSD, you must have an illness that will prevent you from working for at least twelve months. If you first became ill when you were in school, then you would most likely be applying for SSI. If you first became sick when you were working full-time, then SSD would be right for you. What if you were working part-time and going to college part-time? You would most likely qualify for SSI because your job was part-time, but you would need to check this out with someone well acquainted with these services, such as a case manager or the Social Security agency.

You should also know that when you get SSI, in most states you also qualify for Medicaid, the insurance that will pay most of your hospital and medical bills. If you get SSD, there is a waiting period (twenty-four months) before you become eligible for Medicare, another insurance that pays most bills. Sound complicated? It is! But the best way to handle it is to begin by filling out an application that you can get from the Social Security administration office.

Note: The rules for obtaining many of the benefits listed in this chapter vary from state to state and may change over time. Often your local Social Security office can help you with your state's regulations or put you in touch with state offices. If not, check out your state office listed in the back of this book or find your state office on the Web.

Getting the Application

Your treatment manager may already have the application, or you can get it by calling the nearest Social Security office, which should be listed in the phone book under the heading "Government Offices." There is a toll-free phone number you can call from Monday to Friday, between 7:00 a.m. and 7:00 p.m., to get help from a representative: 1–800–772–1213. You can also get information from the Internet at www.ssa.gov.

Filling out the Application

The paperwork is complicated, and it is wise to get help from people who are familiar with filling out applications. Ask your family, case manager, or doctor for assistance. Your doctor will have to fill out the medical section and sign it. If you are applying for SSI, you will have to include a lot of financial information in the application. Your family members may be able to help you with this. If you are applying for SSD, you will not need to disclose your financial situation because it is not required. However, you will be expected to supply information about your work history. The application may seem complicated, but there are many people willing to help you, including workers at your local Social Security office.

ITEMS YOU NEED FOR YOUR SSI APPLICATION

1. Your Social Security number and proof of your age.
2. Information about the home you live in, such as the rent statement, the lease, or the mortgage.
3. Bank books, checkbooks, insurance policy statements, and any other information about how much money you have.
4. The names, addresses, and telephone numbers of your doctors and the hospitals and clinics where you received treatment.
5. Proof of your citizenship or eligible noncitizen status. If you were born in the United States, usually your birth certificate, passport, or army discharge papers will do. If you were born in another country, you will need naturalization papers or proof you were living here legally before 1996.

When documents are required, the agency will want original documents or certified copies. If you are missing any of these items, start the application anyway; the people at the Social Security office or your caseworker will help you find out how to obtain the documents needed.

Eligibility for SSI and SSD

SSI is for people who cannot work and have limited financial resources. If you are over 18 your finances are considered and if you are married, the finances of your spouse are reviewed as well. If you are under 18, your parents' finances are counted for the application. To get SSI you cannot have much money in the bank or in stocks and bonds; currently the limit is $2,000 if you are single and $3,000 if you are married. But the numbers may have changed since this book was printed, so you need to check this out. If you have more money than this, you may be required to "spend down" the balance. This means you will have to pay some of your medical bills with your own money until you get down to the amount you are allowed to keep.

Children and minors (people under the age of eighteen) who are disabled by serious mental illnesses may be eligible to receive Social Security benefits. Social Security Disability Income (SSDI) is available to children and minors when a parent is receiving Social Security benefits or Social

Security Disability benefits. If a parent dies while receiving Social Security benefits, disabled children and minors are entitled to survivor's benefits. Social Security Income (SSI) may be available to children and minors whose family income and resources fall below the level determined by each state. Be sure to have your parent or guardian contact Social Security to get full details for Social Security benefits.

For both SSI and SSD, your doctor must certify that you cannot work because of your illness and that you will not be able to work for at least twelve months. Once you get the application, your doctor will know how to fill it out for you in order for your benefits to start.

If you are not a U.S. citizen, you may still be eligible. If you are a legal immigrant and have been living in the United States since August 22, 1996, you may be eligible if you first became ill after that date. If you came to this country after August 22, 1996, you need to inquire about your eligibility. Call 1–800–772–1213 for the information you need. Your call will be treated confidentially.

ITEMS YOU NEED FOR YOUR SSD APPLICATION

1. Your Social Security number and proof of your age.
2. Names, addresses, and phone numbers of your doctors and the hospitals and clinics where you received treatment.
3. Names of all medications you are taking.
4. Medical records from your doctors, therapists, hospitals, clinics, and caseworkers.
5. Laboratory and test results.
6. A summary of where you worked and what type of work you did.
7. Your most recent W-2 form, or your tax return if you are self-employed.

   You will need original documents or certified copies. If you do not have all these items, you should start the application anyway; the Social Security office will help you find out how to obtain the documents needed.

How Much Money Will You Get?

Once your application is approved, you will get a letter telling you how much money, or benefits, you will be getting. The amount depends on which state you live in and how much money you may already be getting from family members or friends. Your benefits may change from month to month depending on your situation, but usually the amount remains the same. This way you will know how much to expect and be able to plan your expenses.

Some Important Things to Know About Your SSI Check

If you have a bank account, your check will be deposited automatically into it. This is called direct deposit. Many people like direct deposit because the check cannot get lost or damaged. The money is available to you the first of every month. If you do not have an account, you may want to open one so you can have your benefits directly deposited. There may be an easy way to do this if you expect to receive benefits from SSI or SSD. Your case manager will be able to help you, or you may ask the representatives at the Social Security office for assistance. If you do not want direct deposit, you must write this on your application; you will then get a check from the U.S. government on the first of each month, which you will have to cash or deposit. A lost or stolen check can be replaced, but as soon as you know it is missing you will have to call 1–800–772–1213 or visit the Web site, www.ssa.gov, to report it.

There are many things to know that vary from state to state. For example, if you are in the hospital, SSI may continue to pay your rent and other expenses if you are admitted for less than ninety days. When you arrive, tell your doctor or social worker that you are getting SSI. Hospital staff will help you keep your benefits, and you will not need to reapply for SSI. There are special rules for California, Hawaii, Michigan, Vermont, Massachusetts, and New York regarding this procedure. You can find these special rules in the handbook you will receive from Social Security when your benefits are approved. You can get many questions answered online at www.ssa.gov/applyfordisability or by calling 1–800–772–1213.

Special Things to Know for SSI

Keeping good records is really important for both the application process and occasional reviews of your disability status. For example, you need to keep your approval letter (when you get it). For SSI, you need to keep track of your bank books and other bank records and proof of where you live (an electric bill or telephone bill that has been sent to your house).

Every once in a while, staff members from the SSI office will conduct a review, during which they will ask you to show them your bank records and information about your living arrangements. They may also ask your doctor to fill out a form stating how you are doing. The review is done for all people receiving benefits from SSI. There is nothing to be worried about. Your benefits will not be reduced or cut off as long as your assets have not greatly increased and you are not completely well. Having good records makes all of this much easier. But don't worry if you have lost some documents; with a little effort, most can be replaced. Also remember that you may appeal any decision with which you do not agree. The letter telling you of the decision will have instructions on how to appeal.

Special Things to Know for SSD

To be eligible for SSD, you need to have worked at a job that made payments to Social Security out of your gross wages. You can check your pay stubs to see if these payments were made. You also need a certain number of work credits; these are calculated by how much money you made and how long you worked. The people in the Social Security office will be able to tell you your number of work credits and let you know if you are eligible. If you are not eligible for SSD because you do not have enough earned credits, you may want to apply for SSI. Remember, for SSI, your finances will be checked and you must have a very small amount of money and assets like stocks, bonds, and insurance.

Returning to Work or School

Do not be afraid you will lose your benefits if you return to work. Both SSI and SSD provide time to make the adjustment without losing your benefits immediately. If you discover that you began or returned to work prematurely and that you are still ill, you may go right back on SSD and SSI.

On SSD, for the first nine months after returning back to work, you still get your full benefit check regardless of how much money you earn. For the next 36 months the amount you receive from SSD depends on how much money your job pays. You have five years to see if you can keep working. At any time during this period, beginning when you first go back to work, if you find that you cannot continue working, you can go right back on SSD without any waiting period.

If you are receiving SSI and get a job, you may be able to keep your SSI benefits depending on how much you earn. As you earn more, your benefits decrease. The amount you continue to receive in your SSI check varies from state to state. While you are receiving SSI checks, no matter what the amount, you can go back on full SSI if you cannot continue to work. You simply must inform the Social Security office. You do not have to go through the whole reapplication process. If you stop receiving SSI checks because you are earning more than the allowed amount, you still have five years from the date the checks stop to restart your benefits.

197

You may attend an approved vocational rehabilitation program and receive full SSI and SSD benefits.

There are special programs that can help you make the financial transition into school and work. If you are attending school and working, some of your scholarships or wages are not counted as income for SSI. A program called PASS, or "Plan for Achieving Self-Support," allows you to put your earned money aside for education, work-related expenses, vocational training, or starting your own business. You need to notify SSI of your job, your income, and your plans for the future. A counselor from the Social Security office will help you work out a plan. For this program it is important that you keep your pay stubs and a record of your work-related expenses so that your benefits will remain as high as possible for as long as possible. Each state has different rules about benefits for PASS, and the people at your Social Security office can help you apply in your state. If you have questions, you can call 1–800–772–1213 or visit www.ssa.gov. Also, from time to time the rules change. It is always a good idea to check things out at your Social Security office.

Keeping Your Car, House, Condominium, or Co-op

SSI usually does not count your car as part of your assets because they know you may need it to get to appointments, and later on to return to work. If you do not have a car but will require one for work, you may be able to get one without jeopardizing your benefits. This will need to be worked out with your Social Security counselor. If you own your house, condominium, or co-op apartment, you can keep it and still qualify for SSI, but you must continue to pay the mortgage and maintenance bills.

MEDICAL INSURANCE

In addition to private medical insurance, there is government-sponsored insurance: Medicare and Medicaid. In order to fully understand the benefits that these insurances allow, you need to carefully read their benefits explanations, usually provided to you when you become insured. Here is a quick overview of what to expect.

Private Health Insurance

Young adults are sometimes covered by their parents' health insurance, which in most cases allows for health benefits up to age twenty-six. If you fit into this category, you may need to ask your parents how much coverage they have (for example, how many days in the hospital the insurance covers). If you were working when you got sick or if you were in school and had school health insurance, you may need to review the content of those policies. Since this is often written in legal language, you may want to ask for help. Chances are, if you have been hospitalized, the insurance experts at the hospital have already reviewed your benefits and have informed your family about what is covered. But it is good to know this information for yourself so that you can plan ahead. For example, if you know when your benefits will run out, you can plan to apply for SSD or SSI so that you can get Medicare or Medicaid. Understanding how these insurance systems can work for you can relieve the fear that you will not be able to pay your medical bills.

Medicare

Medicare is health insurance from the U.S. government. You become eligible if you receive SSI or SSD for 24 months. As the twenty-fifth month approaches, you will automatically receive a Medicare application in the mail. There are two levels of Medicare. The first, Part A, is free and covers inpatient hospitalizations. The second, Part B, is optional and currently costs about $96 a month, an amount that can be deducted automatically from your SSD or SSI check. Part B covers 80 percent of the costs of doctor and therapist visits outside of the hospital. There is a $135 yearly deductible. Medicare covers most, but not all prescription medications, and there may be a copayment and a fee. Medicare does not pay for most dental care. If Medicare is your only insurance and you need to see a dentist, speak to your case manager or clinician to find out other ways to get dental care. In some states, if a person's finances are very low, the deductible, the copayments, and the monthly fee for Part B are paid by Medicaid.

Sometimes people have both Medicare and Medicaid. This usually happens if you are especially low on funds and there is no one in your household who is working. Questions about Medicare can be answered by calling Social Security at 1–800–772–1213 or Medicare at 1–800–633–4227.

Medicaid

199

Medicaid is a joint program between the states and the federal government to provide health insurance for people who are disabled and/or unable to afford insurance. If you are receiving SSI, you are likely to be covered by Medicaid without any waiting period. In some states, however, this is not true because they have stricter financial requirements for coverage. If this is your situation, your case manager will explain what you need to do to qualify. SSD recipients may or may not be eligible for Medicaid, depending on household income and private insurance from work. If you are not sure about this, you should call your former employer or your state Medicaid office. The offices are listed in your phone book under state government listings. If you call the federal Medicare office at 1–800–633–4227, you can get the number of your state Medicaid office by following the recorded instructions.

MEDICAL BENEFITS FOR CHILDREN AND MINORS

Children and minors (under the age of nineteen) are generally covered by their parents' insurance plans. In some states, if a child/minor develops a permanently disabling illness, the parents' insurance will continue to cover the child/minor for as long as the parents maintain their policy. However, insurance companies do not always advise this option and will require forms filled out well in advance of the date the child/minor's coverage is terminated. Different insurance programs have different rules for when a child/minor is taken off the parents' insurance plan. Those caring for children and young adults should be clear at what age the insurance company will remove children from their parents' coverage. To take advantage of the possibility of keeping parents' insurance, be sure to have family contact the insurance company two to three months before you reach the specified age. Remember, many insurance companies do not notify parents of the possibility of their children staying on their insurance policies and will not honor it if the proper forms are not filed before the young person's coverage is dropped.

Medicaid is available for many children and minors. Benefits vary greatly from state to state, but in general the benefit is based on the family income and assets. Children and minors under the age of eighteen whose families fall below the level of income stipulated by the government can get Medicaid benefits to help pay medical bills. The level of income a family can have to qualify for Medicaid is determined by each state. Once a child/minor turns eighteen, the young person may be considered an adult and be able to get Medicaid based on his/her own income.

Medicare is sometimes available to minors. If a parent receives Medicare while his/her child is a minor, that minor is entitled to Medicare coverage as well. Should the parent die while the child is still a minor, the child is also likely to be entitled to Medicare coverage.

Note: Be sure to check new laws as they are initiated as part of the new health care program.

HOUSING OPTIONS

Many people are able to return to their homes when they are discharged from the hospital. Sometimes things do not work out and a new housing situation must be found. Moving to a new home is one of the top ten stressors for most people. Therefore, it is important to be aware of the alternatives available to you.

You may be able to obtain an apartment on your own, but most people recovering from schizophrenia—or any illness—need some support. Often your case manager can help you find a place to live through various programs in your local area. As you begin to feel better, you may want to make different choices. The important thing is that you take time to adjust to your housing situation and to feel comfortable with yourself in your environment.

THINGS TO CHECK OUT

- Is the neighborhood safe?
- Can I afford the rent and utilities?
- Is there public transportation nearby?
- Can I get to school, work, and my place of treatment?

Government-Sponsored Housing

1. Section *8* housing. This program varies from state to state, but essentially the state contributes to your rent. Sometimes you are allowed to choose your own housing, but sometimes you must live in specified buildings. You have to find out if you qualify and then fill out the application. This can be done at your state housing office, which is sometimes called a Housing Authority. Unfortunately, there are usually not enough Section 8 benefits to go around. It doesn't hurt to get on the waiting list, though. State office staff can give you an idea of how long the wait will be.

2. Supported housing. In supported housing you live alone or with roommates in an apartment and get occasional help from a case manager. The case manager may help you with your budget, planning meals, shopping, and generally managing on your own. Supported housing is part of state programs to help people with schizophrenia and other disabilities live independently in the community.

3. Supportive housing. Supportive housing is more structured than supported housing. It may be in a private home or apartment building, but there are group activities, and you have more time with your case manager. The building management usually works closely with your treatment team.

4. Group homes. Group homes vary in the amount of supervision and help they offer. They typically provide help with daily living skills, medication management, and an overall structure for daily routines. Many group homes are operated by private individuals or organizations licensed by your state. Others are owned and operated by the state.

Daily Activity Requirements for Housing

Most housing facilities require that residents have something constructive to do during the day. This may include attending a day treatment program, going to school full- or part-time, or working. You need not be concerned about having something to do when you first apply. Your social worker or case manager will help you fulfill these requirements by arranging for you to participate in a program.

Resources for Housing Information

National Alliance on Mental Illness (NAMI): 1-800-950-6264; www.nami.org

Mental Health America: 1-800-969-6642; www.nmha.org

Housing Options for People with Mental Illness: www.mentalhealth.org/cmhs

National Resource Center on Homelessness and Mental Illness: www.homelessness.samhsa.gov/

Supplemental Nutrition Assistance Program (SNAP)

202

You may have known about this program when it was called food stamps, but the name has been changed to SNAP by the federal government. Your state may have another name for it, but for all states the way it works is basically the same. The idea is to provide food to people who have a limited amount of money to spend. You may not be ready to think about this now, but at some point you may want to take advantage of SNAP. If you are eligible you receive a card, similar to an ATM card, that allows you to purchase food at most grocery stores. You need to apply for this benefit at your Social Security office; if you are on SSI you may already qualify. If you have SSI, a staff person at Social Security will help you fill out the application and send it to the state SNAP office. If you do not have SSI, you may still qualify. The first step is to get the application from the Social Security office. To learn more about SNAP, go to www.fns.usda.gov/FSP/.

REQUIREMENTS FOR SNAP ELIGIBILITY You must be a citizen of the United States or have legal status as a noncitizen. Eligibility rules are complicated. The best way to determine if you can get SNAP benefits is to apply at your Social Security office. If you are on SSI or have limited financial resources, you may be eligible. The bottom line is that the program can save you money while assuring that you have enough food, so you should apply. Just like in other programs, you can still own a home or an apartment, and a car or truck may not be counted as a resource, depending on how it is used.

ITEMS YOU NEED FOR YOUR SNAP APPLICATION

1. Identification that shows your name and address.
2. Proof of earnings, other income, or SSI benefits. A check stub will do.
3. If you have a child, proof of how much you spend on child care.
4. Utility and rent bills, if you have them.
5. Medical bills for yourself if you are on SSI or SSD.

The SNAP card eliminates the embarrassment of using food stamps. You swipe the card just like any other computerized card. As with all of the other benefits we've discussed, you can be on SNAP only for as long as you need it.

BENEFITS, A COMPLICATED PROCESS

Sometimes getting benefits is unnecessarily complicated. There are so many applications to fill out, records to keep, and offices to visit. But this should not stop you from getting what you need. Here's a tip for making that happen: take one step at a time. First speak with your social worker or case manager; he or she will help you assess your needs. You probably will need some help with your medical bills. You may also need money to live on and even a new place to live.

In this chapter we have outlined some of the benefits that can help you while you are getting well enough to be on your own. You may not require all of these benefits at once, but if you do, take advantage of them. They were put in place for a good reason, to temporarily assist people while they are ill so that they can concentrate on their treatment and not worry about bills. Ask people to help you—your case manager, your doctor, and family members. Accept their help—it's only until you feel better.

When Your Benefits Are Denied

Appeal, appeal, appeal! If you get turned down for any of these benefits, you should appeal. Sometimes large government agencies make mistakes—they may have lost some of your papers or misunderstood your claim. The first thing to do when you get a "denial" letter from the agency to which you applied is to let the government agency know immediately—by phone, by mail, or in person—that you are going to appeal. Then show the letter to your doctor or therapist and get advice about how to proceed. For example, you may need to rewrite a certain section of your application. If you go to the government agency office in person, it is a good idea to bring along a friend or family member so you don't have to go through this process alone. Remember, there are many people ready and willing to help, but they have to know what kind of help you need. Let them know immediately if your request for benefits has been denied.

Mental Health Lawyers and Benefits

There are lawyers who specialize in helping people to get their disability benefits. There are also lawyers who specialize in helping families get appropriate school placements for children with disabilities. Your local legal aid office, NAMI, or your caseworker may be able to help you locate a lawyer who can help if you need to appeal. Legal aid lawyers are especially useful if you do not have funds to pay a lawyer.

Lawyers may also be necessary if parents wish to set up special trust funds for children who have mental illnesses. These trusts make it possible for parents to set aside money in a way that does not affect other benefits they or their children are receiving. Each state has its own rules for setting up trusts. You will need to find a lawyer who knows the rules in your state.

Reminder: Web sites of government agencies may change over time. Similarly, all laws and rules regarding benefits may change as well. Be sure to check with the appropriate sources to get up-to-date benefits information.

17 VOCATIONAL REHABILITATION

Vocational rehabilitation refers to job training and support services. Vocational programs offer places to meet new people and programs that can help you decide what you want to do with your life. In the process, they help you to build your self-confidence and enthusiasm while giving purpose to your life. There are all sorts of resources, many of which are mentioned in this chapter, that can help you move ahead.

WHY VOCATIONAL REHABILITATION?

Anxiety, depression, or unusual thoughts and sensations are generally the symptoms that bring people to a psychiatrist for treatment. Illness may affect life in other important and practical ways as well. It can cause changes in your ability to perform at work, at school, or in social settings. Dealing with these changes is the focus of rehabilitation.

Vocational rehabilitation programs are available for people whose illness makes it difficult for them to choose, get, or keep a job. These programs are available in every state and are funded by the Rehabilitation Services Administration, a unit of the U.S. Department of Education. Services are available through vocational rehabilitation agencies that usually focus on individual needs.

Special contributors: Susanne Mars, M.A., C.R.C., L.P.C.

VOCATIONAL REHABILITATION SERVICES
- **vocational counseling and guidance**
- **assessments to help identify:**
    work skills, abilities, interests
    possible job goals
    services needed to obtain a job
- **training in job skills**
- **support services, including:**
    special transportation
    note takers, interpreters, personal attendants
    books, tools, equipment
    home and worksite modifications
- **job placement assistance:**
    resume preparation
    interview skills training
    on-the-job training
    job coaching

APPLYING FOR SERVICES

To apply for vocational rehabilitation services, begin by calling any of the contact phone numbers listed for the office of vocational rehabilitation in your state (see appendix 2). Inquire about the procedure and get the address of your local office. You may be sent an application to complete prior to your first appointment or you may be given one to complete at the appointment. Ask what documentation you will need to bring with you on your first visit to the vocational rehab office. *Documentation of medical eligibility will be required.* Your doctor or therapist will help you get the papers filled out.

There should be no fee for the initial consultation or for assessments to determine your eligibility for services. However, sponsorship for some services may be based on your income and/or family resources.

A counselor will be assigned to work closely with you and will ask you for information about your background, goals, interests, education, work experience, and physical and mental health, among other things. These questions are asked to help determine the services that will be most helpful to you and to discover the best route to your future employment. Be prepared to participate actively in sharing your ideas, preferences, and concerns about assessment, job training, and future employment with the counselor. This will be a collaborative process in which you and your rehabilitation counselor work together to determine the best plan for your vocational success.

Appeal. If you are dissatisfied with a decision or with the process, you may request a review with a supervisor, a district office manager, or the Client Assistance Program (see appendix 1).

REASONABLE ACCOMMODATIONS ON THE JOB OR AT SCHOOL

People occasionally need "accommodations," which are often minor adjustments to the work environment to allow them to perform effectively at work or school. Provided that an individual meets the qualifications of the job and has the skills to do the job, reasonable accommodations may be requested that address the specific limitations of the disability. For people with physical disabilities, it might be necessary to raise the height of a desk to accommodate a wheelchair; for someone with visual problems, it might be necessary to provide large-print materials.

Reasonable accommodations for someone who has a mental illness serve the same purpose: they allow qualified students and employees to do the best they can by offering special adjustments to the work or school setting. *This does not mean lowering standards of performance or changing entry qualifications for a job or school.* Rather, sensible or practical strategies are applied that do not cause undue hardship to the employer or educator and will help a person with a disability do their job better. It is simply a matter of flexibility about the way the job gets done.

Many people with mental illness are able to perform at work or school without accommodations. For some people, however, mental illness may interfere with their ability to function optimally. Problems with concentration, memory, organization, time management, or relating to other people may make it difficult for them to meet the demands of work or school. Providing sensible strategies in the form of reasonable accommodations can help minimize these problems and increase chances of success.

Before requesting reasonable accommodations, it is helpful to identify the problems in functioning you have encountered since your illness. Your employer or educator is required to provide accommodations only for those limitations that are directly connected to your disability. The next step is to inform the proper people of your need for special accommodations. At work, you will need to tell the human resources department. At school, you must inform the dean of students or the school's disabilities program.

208

Federal legislation known as the Americans with Disabilities Act (ADA) of 1990 is comprehensive civil rights legislation adopted to prohibit discrimination against people with disabilities. This act provides for reasonable accommodations in employment and education. Title I of the ADA provides protection for individuals working for employers with fifteen or more employees. Title II of the ADA provides for reasonable accommodations in educational programs funded by state and local governments.

Your request for reasonable accommodations will be unique to your situation and needs to be evaluated on an individual basis. Therefore, the following lists are meant only as examples of what might be requested, since each person's situation must be evaluated on its own merits.

The following examples are intended to give you an idea of how limitations and reasonable accommodations work together.

Limitation: Difficulty Concentrating

You may be easily distracted, have a short attention span, or have a hard time remembering all the steps of a particular task.

POSSIBLE ACCOMMODATIONS
- take frequent breaks to stretch or walk around
- divide large projects into smaller tasks
- have assignments given one at a time
- request instructions in writing
- engage a tutor to help with study skills

Limitation: The Need to Screen Out Environmental Stimuli

You may be distracted by loud phones, radios, or being in a high-traffic work area.

POSSIBLE ACCOMMODATIONS
- move to less noisy or distracting work or study location
- request volume control on phone or radio

- install high partitions around your desk as sight/sound barriers
- wear headphones that play soothing music

Limitation: Fatigue or Lack of Stamina

Your medication may cause morning fatigue or daytime drowsiness, or you may not have enough energy to work a full day.

POSSIBLE ACCOMMODATIONS

- request a part-time work schedule, flextime, or job sharing
- take mid-day rest breaks
- request exams in sections
- change your work or school schedule to start and end later in order to avoid morning fatigue

For more information about ADA, reasonable accommodations, psychiatric disability, and related topics, see appendix 1.

SUPPORTED EMPLOYMENT

The supported employment model encourages and supports people who have not worked in a while because of their illness to get back into the competitive job market. Working in a government office, at a health agency, or for a business can be therapeutic because it provides a regular routine, spending money, and a place to meet new people. This is how it works. Your case manager or clinician can refer you to a supported employment team where you will meet with counselors to assess your needs. Together, you and the counselors decide on the type of job that would be best for you; they help you every step of the way in getting employment. Once you have the job, you meet with counselors to help you adjust and to resolve any problems that might come up at work. The best thing about this program is that the counselors are there for you when you need them. Of course, you may not need them very often, but it is nice to know that you are supported. For more information ask your case manager or clinician and check out this Web site: http://mentalhealth.samhsa.gov/cmhs/CommunitySupport/toolkits/employment/.

SPECIAL EDUCATION FOR CHILDREN AND MINORS

Special education services are mandated for children with disabilities by the Education for the Handicapped Act (EHA) of 1975; the 1986 amendment for preschool and toddlers; the 1990 amendments (also renaming the law to Individuals with Disabilities Education Act [IDEA]); and the 1997 amendments. Based on the IDEA act and its amendments, children up to the age of twenty-one with disabilities are entitled to appropriate and free education provided by the public education system. Parents of a special needs child can request an Individualized Education Program (IEP) that details the needs and services to be provided. Parents are full participants in the IEP planning and have the right to appeal if they believe the program does not provide appropriate education for their child. Many communities have special education advocates who can help guide parents through the educational planning process. There are also lawyers who specialize in appealing and seeking better educational placements. For example, some communities may not have an appropriate placement, such as a residential school setting, that can provide treatment and education for a young child with schizophrenia. Parents can request that the school go outside its district, even outside its state if need be, to obtain the necessary educational setting.

Appendix 1
Client Assistance Program Directory

Client Assistance Program (CAP) advocates are available to discuss with you any questions or concerns you might have about accessing services for your vocational rehabilitation. If you have questions about your eligibility for vocational services or the development of your vocational goals that cannot be satisfactorily resolved with your vocational counselor or supervisor, the CAP advocates can be helpful.

Alabama
State of Alabama Client Assistance Program   1–800–228–3231
Alaska
Disability Law Center of Alaska   1–800–478–1234 (in state)
Arizona
Arizona Center for Disability Law   1–520–327–9547
                                          1–800–922–1447
Arkansas
Disability Rights Center   1–800–482–1174
California
Client Assistance Program   1–800–952–5544
Colorado
The Legal Center   1–800–288–1376
Connecticut
Office of Protection and Advocacy for Persons with Disabilities
                                          1–800–842–7303 (in state)

Delaware
Client Assistance Program   1–800–640–9336
District of Columbia (Washington, D.C.)
University Legal Services   1–202–547–0198
Florida
Advocacy Center for Persons with Disabilities   1–800–342–0823
Georgia
Client Assistance Program   1–404–373–3116
Hawaii
Protection and Advocacy Agency   1–800–882–1057
                                                                  1–808–949–2922

Idaho
Client Assistance Program   1–800–632–5125 (in state)
Illinois
Illinois Client Assistance Program   1–800–641–3929 (in state)
                                                                  1–217–782–5374
Indiana
Indiana Protection and Advocacy Services   1–800–622–4845
Iowa
Client Assistance Program   1–800–652–4298
Kansas
Client Assistance Program   1–800–432–2326
Kentucky
Client Assistance Program   1–800–633–6283
Louisiana
Advocacy Center for the Elderly and Disabled   1–800–960–7705
                                                                  1–504–522–2337

Maine
Client Assistance Program   1–800–773–7055
                                                                  1–800–452–1948

Maryland
Client Assistance Program   1–800–638–6243
Massachusetts
Client Assistance Program   1–617–727–7440
                                                                  1–800–322–2020

Michigan
Client Assistance Program 1–800–292–4150

1–800–292–5896

Minnesota
Minnesota Disability Law Center 1–800–292–4150   213

1–612–332–1441

Mississippi
Client Assistance Program 1–800–772–4057

Missouri
Missouri Protection and Advocacy Services 1–800–392–8667

Montana
Montana Advocacy Services 1–800–245–4743

Nebraska
Client Assistance Program 1–800–742–7594

Nevada
Client Assistance Program 1–800–633–9879

New Hampshire
Client Assistance Program 1–800–852–3405 (in state)

1–603–271–4175

New Jersey
New Jersey Protection and Advocacy 1–800–922–7233

New Mexico

1–800–432–4682

1–505–256–3100

New York
Client Assistance Program (call collect) 1–800–222–JOBS (5627)

North Carolina
Client Assistance Program 1–800–215–7227 (in state)

North Dakota
Client Assistance Program 1–800–207–6122 (in state)

Ohio
Ohio Legal Rights Service 1–800–282–9181 (in state)

Oklahoma
Client Assistance Program 1–800–522–8224

Oregon
Oregon Advocacy Center 1–800–452–1694

Pennsylvania
Client Assistance Program — 1–888–745–2357
Rhode Island
Rhode Island Disability Law Center — 1–800–733–5332
South Carolina
Client Assistance Program — 1–800–868–0040 (in state)
South Dakota
South Dakota Advocacy Services — 1–800–658–4782 (in state)
Tennessee
Tennessee Protection and Advocacy — 1–800–342–1660
Texas
Client Assistance Program — 1–800–252–9108
Utah
Disability Law Center — 1–800–662–9080
Vermont
Vermont Protection and Advocacy — 1–800–834–7890
Virginia
Client Assistance Program — 1–800–552–3962 (in state)
Washington
Client Assistance Program — 1–800–544–2121 (in state)
West Virginia
West Virginia Advocates — 1–800–950–5250
Wisconsin
Client Assistance Program — 1–800–362–1290 (in state)
Wyoming
Wyoming Protection and Advocacy System — 1–800–821–3091

Appendix 2
Vocational Rehabilitation Directory

The information listed here is presented alphabetically by state. Wherever possible, this directory contains:

- in-state toll-free phone numbers that direct you to local vocational rehab services and/or offices
- local rehab information phone numbers and/or a number for the Client Assistance Program (see appendix 1)
- Web site or Internet addresses where you can access vocational rehab information online; sometimes it is easier to access this information by searching with a Web search engine such as Google to locate sites and contact phone numbers.

State vocational rehab offices may use slightly different names. If you are consulting your local telephone directories for agency listings, consider looking under the following headings:

Division of Vocational Rehabilitation Services
Rehabilitation Services
Jobs Commission
Department of Employment, Training, and Rehabilitation
VESID (Vocational and Educational Services for Individuals with Disabilities)

The state agency that administers the vocational rehabilitation program may be listed in the government section of the phone directory under any of the following:

Department of Human Services
Department of Social Services
Department of Education
Department of Health and Human Services
Department of Human Resources
Department of Economic Security
Department of Labor

Alabama

Alabama Department of Rehabilitation Services

1–800–441–7607
1-334–293–7500
1-334–293–7383 (fax)
www.rehab.state.al.us/Home/default.aspx?url=/Home/Main

Alaska

Alaska Division of Vocational Rehabilitation (see Alaska State Department of Education)

1–800–478–2815 (Juneau branch) (request number of local office)
1–907–465–2814
1–907–465–2856 (fax)
labor.state.ak.us/dvr/home.htm

Arizona

Arizona Rehabilitation Services Administration (see Arizona State Department of Economic Security [DES])

1–800–563–1221 (within Phoenix metro area)
1–602–542–3332 (outside of Phoenix area)
https://egov.azdes.gov/CMSInternet/main.aspx?menu=32&id=1984

Arkansas

Arkansas Division of Vocational Rehabilitation

1–800–330–0632 (Rehab Services administrative offices)
1–501–296–1600
www.arsinfo.org

California

California Department of Rehabilitation

    1–559–445–6011 (Southern Field Office)

    1–530–895–5507 (Northern Field Office)

    1–213–736–3904 (LA/Orange Counties Field Office)

    1–800–952–5544 (Client Assistance Program)

    www.dor.ca.gov

Colorado

Colorado Division of Vocational Rehabilitation

    1–303–444–2816 (Boulder)

    1–303–444–9140 (Boulder fax)

    1–303–772–2612 (Longmont)

    www.cdhs.state.co.us/DVR

Connecticut

Connecticut Bureau of Vocational Rehabilitation (see Connecticut State Department of Social Services)

    1–800–537–2549 (information and referrals) (in Connecticut area)

    www.brs.state.ct.us/programs.htm

Delaware

Delaware Division of Vocational Rehabilitation

    1–800–464–4357 (Delaware Helpline)

    1–302–761–8275

    1–302–761–6611 (fax)

    www.delawareworks.com/dvr/welcome.shtml

District of Columbia (Washington, D.C.)

District of Columbia Department of Human Services

    1–202–442–8663 (vocational rehab information and referrals)

    1–202–442–8400 (intake department)

    dhs.dc.gov/dhs/site/default.asp

Florida

Florida Division of Vocational Rehabilitation (see Florida State Department of Education)

    1–850–488–6210

    www.rehabworks.org

Georgia

Georgia Division of Rehabilitation Services (see Georgia State Department of Human Services)

    1–800–822–9727 (Client Assistance Program)

1–404–486–6331

1—404—232—3910

www.vocrehabga.org

Hawaii

Hawaii Vocational Rehabilitation and Services for the Blind (see Hawaii State Department of Human Services)

1–808–586–5366 or 5368 (administration)

1–808–586–5377 (fax)

hawaiivr.org/main

Idaho

Idaho Division of Vocational Rehabilitation (see Idaho State Board of Education)

1–208–334–3390

1–208–334–5305 (fax)

www.vr.idaho.gov

Illinois

Illinois Department of Human Services

1–800–447—6404

1–800–843–6154 (DHS automated information line)

www.dhs.state.il.us/page.aspx

Indiana

Indiana Division of Disability, Aging, and Rehabilitative Services (see Indiana Family and Social Services Administration)

1–877–282–0964 or 1–877–876–2866 or 1–877–847–9894

1–877–715–5299 or 1–877–396–3271 (regional offices)

www.in.gov/fssa

Iowa

Iowa Division of Vocational Rehabilitation Services

1–800–532–1486 (in Iowa area)

1–515–281–4211

1–515–281–7645 (fax)

www.ivrs.iowa.gov

Kansas

Kansas Department of Social and Rehabilitative Services

1–800–432–2326 (vocational rehab Client Assistance Program)

1–785–296–3959

1–785–296–2173 (fax)

www.srskansas.org

Kentucky

Kentucky Department of Vocational Rehabilitation

1–800–372–7172

1–502–564–4440

ovr.ky.gov

Louisiana

Louisiana Rehabilitation Services (see Louisiana State Department of Social Services)

1–800–737–2958

1–225–925–4131 (state office)

www.dss.state.la.us/index.cfm?md=pagebuilder&tmp=home&nid=12 &pnid=0&pid=72&catid=0

Maine

Maine Bureau of Rehabilitation Services (see Maine State Department of Human Services)

1–800–794–1110

1–207–623–7900

www.maine.gov/rehab/index.shtml

Maryland

Maryland Division of Rehabilitation Services (listed under Maryland State Department of Education)

1–888–554–0334 (Client Services)

1–410–554–9100 or 1–410–554–9385

1–410–554–9412 (fax)

www.dors.state.md.us/dors

Massachusetts

Massachusetts Rehabilitation Commission

1–800–245–6543 (ombudsperson)

1–617–204–3600 or 1–617–204–3603 (ombudsperson)

1–617–727–1354 (fax)

www.mass.gov/?pageID=eohhs2agencylanding&L=4&L0=Home&L 1=Government&L2=Departments+and+Divisions&L3=Massachusetts+ Rehabilitation+Commission&sid=Eeohhs2

Michigan

Michigan Rehabilitation Services Division (see Michigan Department of Career Development)

1–800–292–4150 (Client Assistance Program)

1–800–605–6722 (MJC district offices)

www.michigan.gov/mdcd

Minnesota

Minnesota Division of Rehabilitation Services (see Minnesota State Department of Economic Security)

1–800–657–3858

1–651–259–7114

www.deed.state.mn.us/rehab

Mississippi

Mississippi Department of Rehabilitation Services

1–800–443–1000

1–601–853–5100

www.mdrs.state.ms.us

Missouri

Missouri Division of Vocational Rehabilitation

1–877–222–8963

1–573–751–3251

1–573–751–1441 (fax)

dese.mo.gov/vr

Montana

Montana Department of Public Health and Human Services

1–888–279–7528 (Missoula disability services division)

1–888–279–7527 (Great Falls disability services division)

1–888–279–7532 (Billings disability services division)

1–888–279–7531 (Butte disability services division)

www.dphhs.mt.gov

Nebraska

Nebraska Vocational Rehabilitation (see Nebraska State Department of Education)

1–800–742–7594 (hotline for disability services)

1–877–637–3422

1–402–471–3644 (Vocational Rehab state office)

www.vocrehab.state.ne.us

Nevada

Nevada Rehabilitation Division

1–800–633–9879 (Client Assistance Program)

1–775–684–4070 (Northern Nevada Vocational Rehab)

1–775–423–6568 (Rural Nevada Vocational Rehab)

1–702–486–5230 (Southern Nevada Vocational Rehab)

detr.state.nv.us/rehab/reh_index.htm

New Hampshire

New Hampshire Department of Health and Human Services

1–800–299–1647 (Vocational Rehab) (a division of the Department of Education) (in New Hampshire area)

1–603–271–3471

www.dhhs.state.nh.us/DHHS/DHHS_SITE/default.htm

New Jersey

New Jersey Division of Vocational Rehabilitation Services

1–609–292–5987

lwd.dol.state.nj.us/labor/dvrs/DVRIndex.html

New Mexico

New Mexico Division of Vocational Rehabilitation

1–800–224–7005

1–505–954–8500

1–505–954–8562 (fax)

www.dvrgetsjobs.com/index/index.aspx

New York

New York VESID (see New York State Department of Education)

1–800–222–JOBS (1–800–222–5627)

www.vesid.nysed.gov

North Carolina

North Carolina Division of Vocational Rehabilitation (see North Carolina State Department of Health and Human Services)

1–800–662–7030 (care line information and referral) (request DVR representative)

1–800–689–9030

1–919–855–3579

dvr.dhhs.state.nc.us

North Dakota

1–800–472–2622 (North Dakota Department of Human Services)

1–800–755–2745 (vocational rehab information and referral)

www.nd.gov/dhs

Ohio

Ohio Rehabilitation Services Commission

1–800–282–4536

1–614–438–1200

1–614–438–1257 (fax)

www.rsc.state.oh.us/default.aspx

Oklahoma

Oklahoma Department of Rehabilitation Services

1–800–845–8476 (in Ohio area)

1–405–951–3400

1–405–951–3529 (fax)

www.okrehab.org

Oregon

Oregon Vocational Rehabilitation Division (see Oregon State Department of Human Resources)

1–503–945–5944

www.oregon.gov/DHS/vr

Pennsylvania

Pennsylvania Office of Vocational Rehabilitation

1–800–442–6351 (central administrative office) (in Pennsylvania area)

1–717–787–5244

www.nepacil.org/OVR.htm

Rhode Island

Rhode Island Office of Rehabilitation Services (see Island State Department of Human Services)

1–800–752–8088 ext. 2300

1–401–421–7005

1–401–222–3574 (fax)

www.ors.ri.gov

South Carolina

South Carolina Department of Vocational Rehabilitation

1–803–896–6500

www.scvrd.net/

South Dakota

South Dakota Division of Rehabilitation Services (see South Dakota State Department of Human Services)

1–800–265–9684 (request a division of rehab services for information)

1–605–773–5990
1–605–773–5483 (fax)
dhs.sd.gov/drs

Tennessee

Tennessee Division of Rehabilitation Services (see Tennessee State
Department of Human Services)

1–615–313–4891 (vocational rehab main office)
www.state.tn.us/humanserv

Texas

Texas Rehabilitation Commission

1–800–628–5115 or 512–424–4000 (general information)
1–800–252–9108 (Client Assistance Program)
www.dars.state.tx.us

Utah

Utah Office of Rehabilitation

1–800–473 7530 (Rehab Services administrative office)
1–801–538 7530
1–801–538 7522 (fax)
www.usor.utah.gov

Vermont

Vermont Vocational Rehabilitation Division

1–800–361–1239 (in Vermont area)
1–802–241–2186 (Vocational Rehabilitation Director)
1–802–241–3359 (fax)
vocrehab.vermont.gov

Virginia

Virginia Department of Rehabilitative Services

1–800–552–5019
www.vadrs.org

Washington

Washington Division of Vocational Rehabilitation

1–800–637–5627 (Division of Vocational Rehab)
1–800–737–0617 (Department of Health and Rehabilitative Services)
(in Washington area)
1–360–438–8007 (fax)
www.dshs.wa.gov/dvr

West Virginia

West Virginia Division of Rehabilitation Services (see West Virginia State Department of Education and the Arts)

    1–800–642–8207 (rehab information and local offices)

    1–800–950–5250 (Client Assistance Program)

    www.wvdrs.org

Wisconsin

Wisconsin Division of Vocational Rehabilitation

    1–800–442–3477 (press zero for DVR receptionist)

    dwd.wisconsin.gov/dvr

Wyoming

Wyoming Vocational Rehabilitation Division (see Wyoming State Department of Employment)

    1–307–777–7389 (Vocational Rehab Division Administrator)

    1–307–777–5939 (fax)

    www.wyomingworkforce.org/vr

━━

Bazelon Center for Mental Health Law

Phone (not toll-free): 1–202–467–5730

www.bazelon.org

E-mail: webmaster@bazelon.org

    The Judge David L. Bazelon Center for Mental Health Law is a leader in legal advocacy for people with mental illnesses. They are not able to help with individual requests, but they are a good source of written legal information. For individual requests look for your state's protection and advocacy agency on the NAPAS Web site, listed below.

Center for Mental Health Services—Housing Options

Toll-free number: 1–800–789–2647

www.mentalhealth.org/cmhs

E-mail: ken@mentalhealth.org

    This organization provides information on a number of issues for people with mental illness, including help with finding housing. By calling their phone number or using their Web site, you can find local agencies that will help you with housing needs. This agency provides similar services as the National Resource Center on Homelessness and Mental Illness.

NAMI—National Alliance for the Mentally Ill

Toll-free number: 1–800–950–NAMI (6264)

www.nami.org

NAMI is a nonprofit, grassroots, self-help, support, and advocacy organization of consumers, families, and friends of people with mental illness such as schizophrenia, major depression, bipolar disorder, obsessive-compulsive disorder, and anxiety disorders. Working at national, state, and local levels, NAMI provides education about brain disorders, supports increased funding for research, and advocates for adequate health insurance, housing, rehabilitation, and jobs for people with psychiatric illnesses.

The *Family-to-Family Education Program* is a free twelve-week course for family caregivers of individuals with severe mental illness.

NARSAD—The Brain and Behavioral Research Fund

Toll-free number: 1–800–829–8289; or (not toll-free) 1–516–829–0091

www.narsad.org

NARSAD is a donor-supported research organization funding research for psychiatric illnesses. This organization has a useful Web site for learning about schizophrenia research.

National Association of Protection and Advocacy (NAPAS)

Phone (not toll-free): 1–202–408–9514

www.napas.org

The National Association of Protection and Advocacy keeps track of a number of legal and policy issues that affect people with disabilities, including on-the-job rights and discrimination in all areas. By calling their phone number or sending them e-mail, you will be connected to your state office of protection and advocacy. For example, if you are interested in writing an advance psychiatric directive, the state office can provide guidance on how to proceed. Since the laws in each state are slightly different, for most matters it is important that legal issues are addressed on the state level.

National Clearinghouse for Alcohol and Drug Abuse

Toll-free number: 1–800–729–6686 (to speak to a live person, listen carefully to menu)

www.samhsa.gov and www.health.org

The National Clearinghouse runs a telephone hotline where you can request information about drug abuse to be mailed to you; your address is kept confidential. It will also refer callers to local treatment agencies without requesting names or addresses. The Web site provides links to information sources and referrals. This service is part of the Substance Abuse and Mental Health Services Administration (SAMHSA) and is geared to helping people with mental illness and substance abuse.

National Depressive and Manic-Depressive Association

Toll-free number: 1–800–826–3632

www.ndmda.org

The National Depressive and Manic-Depressive Association provides information about depression and mania upon request. The organization also refers consumers and family members to support groups located throughout the United States. Additional information is available on their Web site.

National Institute of Mental Health (NIMH)

Toll-free number:1–866–615–6464; local number 301–443–4513

www.nimh.nih.gov/index.shtml

E-mail: nimhinfo@nih.gov

The NIMH is a branch of the National Institutes of Health. Its mission is to transform "the understanding and treatment of mental illness through research." This site offers a wealth of information, including free booklets, online videos, the latest research initiatives, and what is new in research and treatment. You can also get information on enrolling in one of the NIMH's research studies if this interests you.

National Mental Health Consumer's Self-Help Clearinghouse

Toll-free number: 1–800–553–4KEY (4539)

www.mhselfhelp.org

This clearinghouse provides self-help resource information geared toward meeting the individual and group needs of mental health consumers. It provides advocacy, listings of publications, on-site consultations, training, and educational events.

National Mental Health Association

Toll-free number: 1–800–969-NMHA (6642)

www.nmha.org

The National Mental Health Association provides free information on more than 200 mental health topics, referrals to mental health providers, and a directory of local mental health associations. NMHA also advocates to remove the stigma of mental illness.

National Resource Center on Homelessness and Mental Illness

Toll-free number: 1–800–444–7415

E-mail: nrc@prainc.com

The National Resource Center on Homelessness and Mental Illness provides information about homelessness and gives referrals to local agencies that can help people find a place to live. You may also e-mail your questions about housing options.

North American Society for Childhood-Onset Schizophrenia (NASCOS)

www.nascos.org

NASCOS is an organization of parents with younger children who have schizophrenia. This organization can provide support and educational resources to families of young children with schizophrenia.

Schizophrenia Society of Canada

Toll-free number (in Canada): 1–800–263–5545

www.schizophrenia.ca

The Schizophrenia Society of Canada provides information in English and French and referrals to provincial support and information groups in Canada. Membership in the national organization is free, but there may be a small fee for membership in local groups. Joining entitles members to the national newsletter, local news, and social events in the provinces throughout Canada.

Schizophrenia.com

www.schizophrenia.com

Schizophrenia.com is a nonprofit organization that calls itself a "Web community." It has a friendly Web site with good resources and information for people with schizophrenia.

Self-Help Sourcebook

www.mentalhelp.net/selfhelp

This site helps you locate mental health self-help groups in your community in the United States and Canada.

Social Security Administration

Toll-free number: 1–800–772–1213

www.ssa.gov

The Social Security Administration is the U.S. government office that manages and distributes information and pamphlets about SSI, SSD, and Medicare. Local offices have the applications and forms to fill out, and are listed in the phone book, usually in the U.S. government section. You can also find the address and the business hours of your local office by calling the toll-free number or visiting the Web site. Information about Medicaid is provided by your state's Medicaid offices, usually listed in the state government section of your phone book, or you can call Medicare at 1–800–633–4227.

ADDITIONAL WEB SITES OF INTEREST

GOVERNMENT AGENCIES

- Every state has an Office or Department of Mental Health, with contact information available on the Web.
- Center for Mental Health Services, Knowledge Exchange Network (Substance Abuse and Mental Health Services Administration, U.S. Department of Health and Human Services): www.mentalhealth.org
- National Institute on Drug Abuse (National Institutes of Health): www.nida.nih.gov
- National Institute of Mental Health (National Institutes of Health): www.nimh.nih.gov/index.shtml
- Substance Abuse and Mental Health Services Administration: www.samhsa.gov
- Some states have an Office of Mental Retardation and Developmental Disabilities, with contact information available on the Web.

PROFESSIONAL ORGANIZATIONS

American Psychiatric Association: www.psych.org

American Academy of Psychiatry and Law: www.aapl.org

American Academy of Child and Adolescent Psychiatry: www.aacap. org

American Psychological Association: www.apa.org

American Association for Correctional Psychology: www.eaacp.org

MENTAL HEALTH ORGANIZATIONS

National Mental Health Association: www.nmha.org

State Mental Health Associations can be found in all states, with contact information available on the Web.

MEDICATION ASSISTANCE PROGRAMS

- NeedyMeds.com is a nonprofit organization that provides an extensive Web site filled with information, including a listing of patient assistance programs sponsored by drug companies.
- Partnership for Prescription Assistance is sponsored by pharmaceutical research companies. The organization's mission is to help those who cannot afford prescription medications and do not have insurance to cover medication. Call toll free, 1-888-477-2669, or visit their site, www.pparx.org.
- Pharmaceutical companies may offer medication assistance directly. Check Web sites or get help from you doctor or case manager.

MENTAL HEALTH RESEARCH TRIALS

Clinical research trials for schizophrenia and many other illnesses are conducted around the country. A listing of research trials can be found at www.clinicaltrials.gov

USING THE INTERNET TO GET THE INFORMATION YOU NEED

Using the Internet is a great opportunity to get useful and up-to-date information about schizophrenia, substance abuse, and other subjects that you may be interested in.

A word of caution: Reliable Web sites are the way to go. Only there will you get information that is truly useful. Because the Internet is open for anyone to post anything, some information can be misleading and wrong. When surfing the Web, use your judgment to decide if a site seems legitimate or not. Web sites that appear to be professional and official are generally the ones you want to use. Here are a few reliable sites that can give you a general idea of what a good Web site looks like:

www.nimh.nih.gov

231

www.schizophrenia.com

www.nami.org

And Then There Is Blogging . . .

Blogs are another useful Internet tool that you might find helpful and even fun. Here are a few things about blogs that are important to know:

- Blogs are a way to connect with others who have the same interests as you.
- Blogs are Web sites where people post information or personal experiences and thoughts on any given topic.
- Blogs for schizophrenia usually consist of personal stories and experiences with schizophrenia.
- You can comment on other people's blogs if you go to a person's Web site. You can write about your own feelings, experiences, or opinions.
- You also have the option of creating your very own blog, where you can share your own experiences.
- Important! Sometimes you can get useful information from other bloggers, but because everyone is different, what is right for someone else may not be what you need.
- In general, it is best not to rely on any information provided on blogs because it may not be accurate.

Remember, blogs are only personal opinions and experiences from others, so steer away from anything that makes you feel uncomfortable. If you have a question about something you see on a blog, don't keep it to yourself—talk to your therapist or doctor.

On the positive side, blogs are a great way to connect to others who may be going through similar experiences. You can both gain and give support on subjects that you share in common. Want to see some blogs? Go to www.schizophrenia.com for a list of some popular blogs. There is even a link that shows you how to set up one for yourself. Happy and safe blogging!

Remember that not everything you read on the Web is accurate. When using the Internet to find information, look for sites associated with government, educational institutions, and legitimate organizations.

PUBLICATIONS AND VIDEOS OF INTEREST

Schizophrenia

Breakthroughs in Antipsychotic Medications: A Guide for Consumers, Families and Clinicians, by Peter Weiden, Patricia L. Scheifler, Ronald J. Diamond, Rut Ross (NAMI, 1999).

Getting Your Life Back Together When You Have Schizophrenia, by Roberta Temes (New Harbinger, 2002).

Living with Schizophrenia (DVD) (Guilford Press, 2006).

Me, Myself, and Them: A Firsthand Account of One Young Person's Experience with Schizophrenia, by Kurt Snyder, Raquel E. Gur, and Linda Wasmer Andrews (Oxford University Press, 2007).

Schizophrenia for Dummies, by Jerome Levine and Irene S. Levine (Wiley, 2009).

Surviving Schizophrenia: A Manual for Families, Patients, and Providers, by E. Fuller Torrey (Harper, 2006).

SZ Schizophrenia Digest. www.schizophreniadigest.com

The Quiet Room: A Journey Out of the Torment of Madness, by Lori Schiller and Amanda Bennett (Grand Central Publishing, 1996).

Understanding Mental Illness and Schizophrenia (DVD) (Information Television Network, 2006).

Drug Addiction

The Dual Diagnosis Recovery Sourcebook: A Physical, Mental, and Spiritual Approach to Addiction with an Emotional Disorder, by Dennis Ortman (McGraw-Hill, 2001).

How to Quit Drugs for Good: A Complete Self-Help Guide, by Jerry Dorsman (Three Rivers Press, 1998).

Index